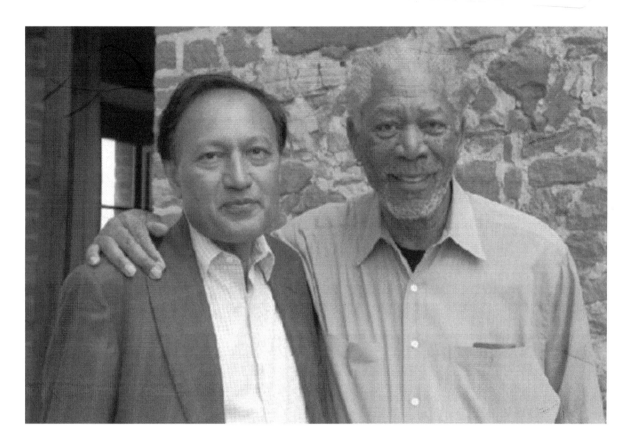

I promise you, this is amazing stuff.

Morgan Freeman

# About Dr Mosaraf Ali

Mosaraf Ali is a pioneer in integrated medicine. He blends the science of conventional medicine with elements of traditional systems such as Herbal Medicine, Ayurveda and Unani to produce a unique, safe and highly effective method of healthcare. His philosophy is based on the Hippocratic Principles, which state that we all have an innate healing power that can cure most ailments and restore well-being.

Dr. Ali's simple Lifestyle Programme of diet, massage, yoga and natural supplements nurtures this healing power. It has been developed over 28 years of clinical experience, working with patients from all walks of life, from the most disadvantaged to celebrities and royalty.

Dr. Ali has written seven books and wrote a health column for six years in *The Mail* on Sunday and in *Top Santé* magazine. He trains doctors in integrated medicine, has carried out research into the effects of his massage therapy in stroke rehabilitation, speaks regularly at conferences around the world and heads the clinical spa at Castel Monastero in Tuscany, Italy, as well as practising from his central London clinic. He also has a charity clinic in a village in the Indian Himalayas, providing free medical care to over 50,000 needy people.

Published in Great Britain 2011 and in the United States 2011

Published by Sugar and Spice Resources Limited
PO Box 182 Channel House
Forest Lane St. Peter Port Guernsey GY1 4HL
Email: info@neckconnection.com
Website: www.neckconnection.com
www.drmali.com


Edited by Ken Bridgewater and Azeem Ali

ISBN: 978-0-9569028-4-9

*To*
*His Majesty*
*Sultan Qaboos*
*Bin Said Al Said,*
*The Sultanate of Oman*

# Contents

## Part 3 – The Solution

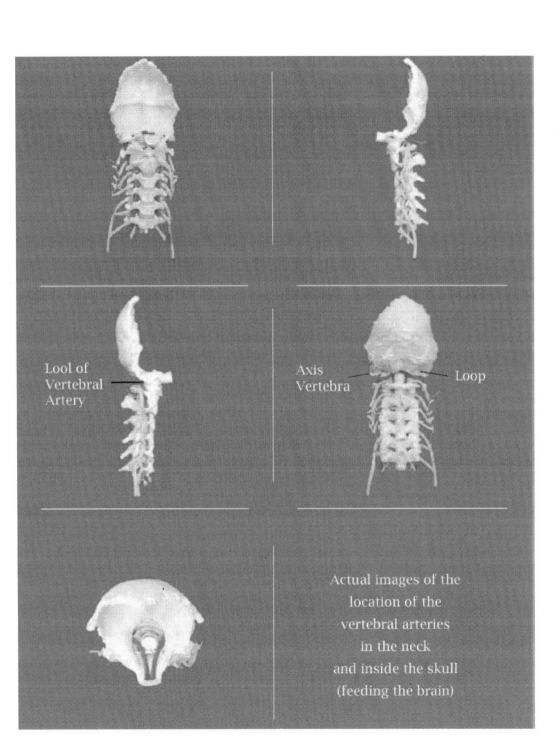

Lool of
Vertebral
Artery

Axis
Vertebra

Loop

Actual images of the
location of the
vertebral arteries
in the neck
and inside the skull
(feeding the brain)

# Part 1 - The Problem

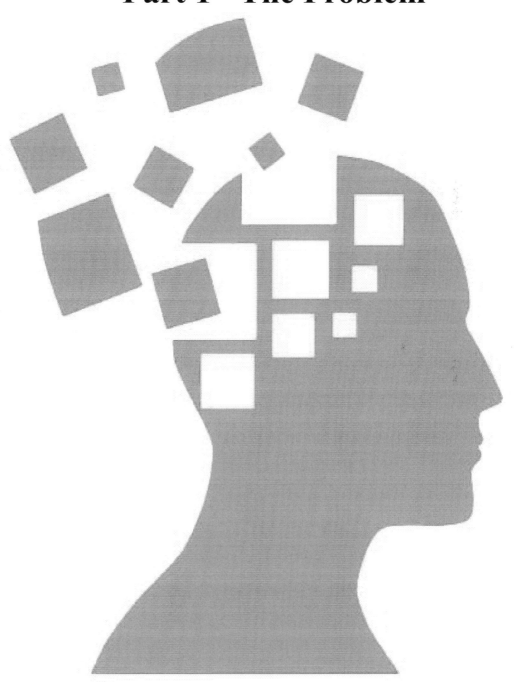

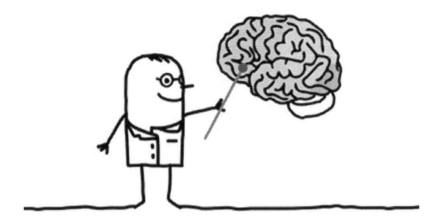

*Then, something happened and my attitude towards medicine changed completely – you could almost say a 'EUREKA' moment – when I found the secret of spontaneous and innate healing ...*

Traditionally a sharp blow to the neck can be fatal. No other part of the body is so vulnerable. This concept precedes all the hangings, garrotting and strangling of our modern era. During the classical era, the Roman Emperor Caligula allegedly said "Oh if the people had but one neck" namely a shared vulnerability so he could slay them all with one stroke. Over the years the neck has appeared in many phrases emphasising its weakness: if you "stick your neck out" you offer your most vulnerable part to your enemy or if you keep it strong by being "stiff necked" or "brass necked" you are more secure. You "get it in the neck" when you receive punishment or reprimand. If you disappear to some far off "neck of the woods" you make yourself less traceable so reducing your vulnerability. But you can express pride or self-confidence with "chin up" and if you treat it gently it can be a source of well-being or pleasure. As Frank Sinatra put it so succinctly to Debbie Reynolds in the Tender Trap "Let's neck". This book, however, is not so concerned with the lethality of blows to the neck as to a whole host of apparently unrelated symptoms, following lesser traumas, which are less identifiable and frequently misdiagnosed. We will consider both together – "neck and neck".

# Chapter 1 – The Revelation

## My Revelation

How did my fascination for the neck arise? After completion of my medical studies and post graduation in 1982 in Moscow, I worked in Delhi for six years and built-up a very successful practice in Integrated Medicine. I combined my medical knowledge and experience with what I had learnt in Traditional and Complementary Medicine. In those days I used conventional or allopathic medicine to treat acute conditions, such as flu, severe migraine, high blood pressure, diarrhoea etc For treatment of chronic backache, fatigue, IBS, asthma etc, I used acupuncture, herbal remedies (both Ayurveda and Unani), homeopathy, yoga and some massage.

Initially, people were sceptical about this combination of different types of medicine, but as stories and success began to spread, my practice grew. Then, something happened and my attitude towards medicine changed completely – you could almost say a 'EUREKA' moment – when I found the secret of spontaneous and innate healing.

I was invited to Bangkok at short notice to see someone who had mysteriously slipped into a coma. My flight left Delhi at 2AM and I landed just under four hours later. I was totally exhausted. The man who came to meet me wanted me to go directly to the hospital as the patient was in a critical condition. However, I needed a few hours sleep and time to prepare to treat him. He then offered to take me somewhere where I could have quick treatment myself.

I was taken to someone's home near a temple. I was shown into a basement room and asked to lie down. He gently grabbed my neck, but what followed was unbelievably painful. He began to press hard and found some sore spots in the neck, occiput and shoulders. He stretched my neck, twisted it sideways and gave it a sudden jerk to crack my displaced joints. It was a form of manipulation used, I knew, by chiropractors and osteopaths. I then felt a 'gush' of blood into the head and I had a tingling sensation in my brain. The dimly lit room seemed brighter and there wasn't a slightest hint of exhaustion left in my body; I felt instantly 'rejuvenated'. 'What a strange experience!' I thought.

I then went straight to the hospital, feeling fresh, to give the patient some acupuncture. I also decided to massage his neck and shoulders, as I was convinced that the neck treatment could stimulate the brain – I was already aware of some acupuncture points in the neck, which help to combat headaches and dizziness. However, as he was on a ventilator, it was difficult to stretch and manipulate the area.

As I carried out my treatment, the patient's eyelids flickered and there was some movement in his toes. I continued to use this therapy, three times a day – it was total guesswork at this point, as I had never used this technique before. I had also brought some powder of pearl and drops containing musk which are traditional remedies for weakened patients and are known to stimulate the nervous system and increase the chance of revival? On the third day, success came when the patient opened his eyes and the ventilator was removed. Further treatment followed and the patient recovered. The doctors believed it was a case of spontaneous recovery, whilst I was totally convinced that the acupressure, neck massage and stimulation of the nervous system did the trick.

## Follow up

I then decided to explore further. I had heard that in a Naturopathy centre at Phillaur in the Punjab, a northern Indian state, hot water was used to stimulate the neck and spine of most patients once a day. Hot water was poured down the neck and spine from an aluminium kettle with a long nozzle. I then went to Jiwan Nagar in Haryana, some four hours drive from Delhi, where I used to hold free medical camps for poor villagers twice a month.

During one of my visits, I was shown a bed with rollers. The patient lay on the bed, was grabbed by the legs and their neck and upper back were rolled up and down the bed. This treatment was used to massage the neck and shoulder and to stimulate the nerves. Patients with chronic ailments, such as headaches, fatigue, backache, and various nervous disorders were treated with the 'Rolling technique' with some success. 'Why the neck and shoulder?' I wondered.

With my inquisitive and analytical brain ticking, I opened my Anatomy Atlas and began to study the pictures of the neck and back.

I realised that one pair of the arteries and veins in the neck were hidden away in a canal that runs on either side of the neck vertebrae. This pair of canals is formed by the lateral holes in the wings of the neck vertebrae and by thick sheets of fibrous tissue. My initial question was: 'why has Nature protected these arteries so well?' No other blood vessels were so well treated – except for those in the heart, which beats constantly so the risk of pressure on vital arteries is high. There had to be a reason why they had received such strong protection from the firm sheath of fibrous tissue. The logical answer was: these blood vessels must be extremely vital for the very existence of the body.

I began to trace these arteries, which are called Vertebral Arteries, to the brain. I could not believe what I discovered. These arteries supplied blood to the subconscious part of the brain which carries out all the 'automatic 'or 'unconscious' functions of the body. Without this part of the brain, nothing in the body can function. Moreover, it is the most ancient part of the brain in evolution, if we are able to believe in that. Our very existence depends on the blood supplied through these arteries and the waste drained down via the corresponding veins to and from the Subconscious Brain.

The logic is simple. The Conscious Brain appeared later in the evolutionary history, so the arteries that feed it also developed later. Similarly, if cancer develops somewhere in the body, a new network of blood vessels develops to feed it. The blood vessels that developed to feed the Conscious Brain predominantly are known as the Carotid Arteries, which are located in the front of the neck and are only protected by muscles; no canals or tubes protect them. They are freestanding.

All vertebrates have Vertebral Arteries, but only mammals (human, monkeys, elephants, lions, dogs etc) are gifted with the Conscious or Cortical Brain, have Carotid Arteries. Nature has made this clear-cut distinction, based upon the type of nervous or mental activities they carry out. At this point, therefore, I must explain what the Conscious and Subconscious brain does.

# Chapter 2 – The Brain

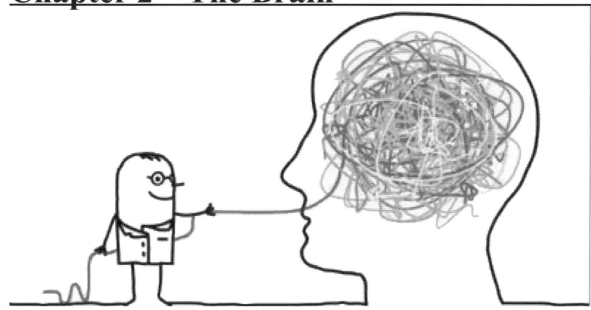

*Today, the art of logic is replaced by the science of physics, mathematics and chemistry to prove things. However, the Latin word for 'to prove' is 'experiri' to which the words 'experience' and 'experiment' are both related. In other words proof can be by experiment (science) or by experience (logic). It is therefore a mistake to replace one with the other; we still depend heavily on both…*

The brain is a controversial subject, as the very existence of the subconscious, termed as 'involuntary', 'automatic' or 'unconscious' functions of the brain, is poorly defined or understood by science. Here one has to rely on logic, the age-old method of proving and analyzing things used so brilliantly by the great philosophers such as Aristotle, Plato, and Socrates. Today, the art of logic is replaced by the science of physics, mathematics and chemistry to prove things. However, the Latin word for 'to prove" is 'experiri' to which the words 'experience' and 'experiment' are both related. In other words proof can be by experiment (science) or by experience (logic). It is therefore a mistake to replace one with the other; we still depend heavily on both.

# The Two Brains: Conscious and Subconscious

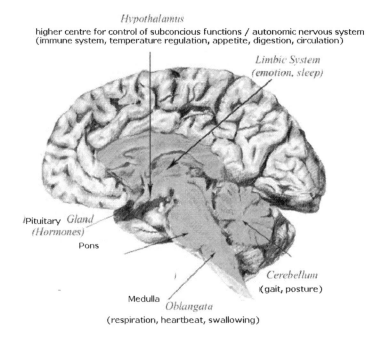

Figure (B)

(Section of the brain showing the subconscious brain. Blue coloured portion is subconscious brain)

# 1. The Conscious Brain

This is known as the Cortical Brain and forms the superficial or outer layers, of the brain. It makes decisions, analyses, makes deductions, uses logic, makes voluntary movements; senses pain, heat, touch, vision, hearing, smell etc; stores long-term memory, and above all, is responsible for our intellectual function- thinking. The Subconscious Brain or Unconscious Brain deals with everything else. It regulates hormones; maintains body temperature; controls heartbeat, breathing, digestion, appetite, balance, gait, posture, sexual functioning, sleep, energy levels, the immune system, emotions, short-term memory etc These subconscious functions of the brain are complicated and are beyond our voluntary decisions or Will, for any effective control. For example, if you walk into a sauna with an extremely high temperature, within seconds of your being there the body's temperature control 'automatically' reacts by raising the heart rate; opening up the pores to secrete sweat; dilating blood vessels etc. The adaptive process cannot be regulated by our conscious brain, which generally works more slowly. If you touch a thorn on a rose stem and, in a quick reflex action, pull your hand away, you do so even before you feel the pain, which is a conscious action. The Conscious Brain cannot have the capacity to analyze the exact component of food; both the quantity and chemical structure of the ingested matter. The Subconscious Brain does that for us and achieves perfect digestion; the absorption of useful matter and elimination of waste. Thus, Nature made a unique system of control within the body that helps to sustain life and regulate all its functions.

Certain functions of the body are both consciously (voluntarily) and/or unconsciously (involuntarily)39 controlled. We know breathing is involuntary, taking place at the rate of 16 breaths per minute. Yet, it can be voluntarily controlled. Pearl divers hold their breath for 7-10 minutes. Yoga and meditation involve breath control. Singing and playing wind instruments require voluntary control of the breath for the desired effect. Similarly, our erect posture can be changed voluntarily. Our skills begin by being a voluntary action but with some practice soon become involuntary or part of our unconscious. Standing, walking, riding a bicycle, driving, writing, playing a musical instrument all start off by voluntarily exercising certain groups of muscles and then with some training, the control becomes automatic or involuntary. We do not need to 'use our brain' most of the time. Both speech and writing are perfect examples where thoughts are translated into movement involuntarily and instantly.

One can continue to be alive without the conscious brain, as its role is not entirely vital. Lobotomy, a disgusting operation performed on psychologically affected people, proves the point. When the frontal lobe of the cortical brain is removed, the person continues to live normally, except that he or she cannot think, as the intellectual functions no longer exist.

Diseases that affect the Cortical Brain do not affect life processes. Superficial brain haemorrhage, stroke, benign tumours, coma etc affect the conscious brain and so the heartbeat, breathing and the vital symptoms continue, as these centres are not affected. Somewhere in the world I heard, a man in coma had been kept alive for 22 years with a life-support machine.

A clot travelling through the vertebral arterial network is fatal in a majority of cases. The clot will plug one or the other smaller arteries cutting off the blood supply to vital centres of the brain. Thus, the vertebral arteries feeding the subconscious brain are vital to the person's survival.

In a very crude way, we can see the effect of Halal or Kosher methods of slaughtering animals. When the carotid arteries of the neck are severed by this method, the conscious brain dies but, because the vertebral arteries remains untouched, the subconscious brain continues to function for a few minutes. The heart beats and so the circulation of blood continues. This helps to flush out blood from the flesh as the bleeding through the carotid arteries continues. The meat is 'freed' from toxins in the blood and is supposedly tastier than the flesh of animals killed instantly. I must stress I intend no disrespect to the practitioners by using this as an example.

Just as the lungs and heart are protected by the ribcage, the brain, which is the most important and delicate organ of the body, is protected by a tough skull. There are also tough membranes that lie beneath the skull. Finally, there is fluid that bathes the outer and inner surface of the brain. In fact, the brain is buoyant in this fluid so, if the head moves, the brain (like a buoy), remains relatively static and its surface don't collide with the skull. The brain is kept safe, while its owner is jumping, running, skipping etc, by this fluid, known as Cerebro Spinal Fluid (CSF).

The Subconscious Brain lies beneath the thick layer of the Cortical or Conscious Brain. Thus, in an accident when the outer surface is shaken-up, one suffers concussion and looses consciousness. The heart and lungs, whose control centres are located deep in the subconscious brain, often remain unaffected and continue to function. If you imagine a cauliflower or broccoli, the outer flower is the cortical or conscious brain and the stalks or stems, in the centre represent the subconscious brain. These stalks are tougher; more resilient and are also protected by the flower on top (stalks have fibres which are tough).

## 2. The Subconscious Brain

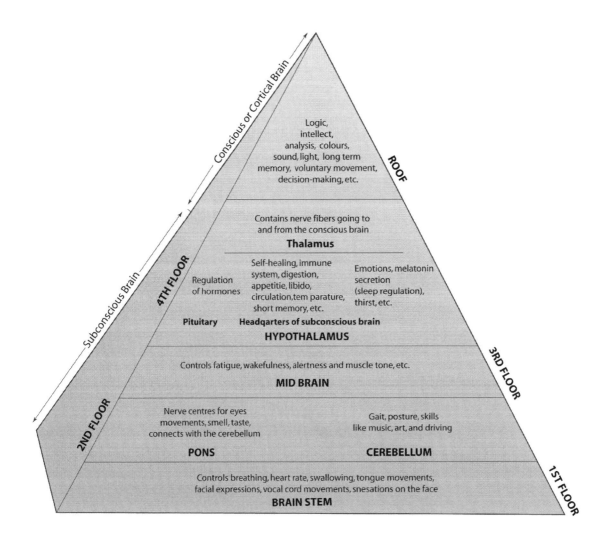

Figure (C)

I do not intend to go into the detailed anatomy of the Subconscious Brain but some description is necessary to explain where things are located. If you look at the brain in a standing position, it is like a four storey building. The roof consists of the Cortical or Conscious Brain, with the higher centres of intellect: logic, voluntary movements, analysis of pain, light, sound, colour, decision making etc the fourth floor (Diencaphalon) consists of a split level flat. The upper portion (Thalamus) houses all the nerve fibres or cables, going to and from the Cortical Brain. The lower portion, called the Hypothalamus, which is below the Thalamus, houses the headquarters of the Subconscious Brain. This is the command centre, from where instructions are given to all the automatic or involuntary functions of the body. This is also the intelligence centre, which receives and analyses the goings-on in the body. The passage of food through the intestines; heart rate; breathing; the emotional state of the body; hormone levels etc are all controlled from here. The Hypothalamus is also the appetite centre; the thermostat or body temperature regulator; circulation centre; water retention centre; short-term memory; sexual urge (libido and orgasm); emotional controls; labour; milk production; stomach acid secretion; adaptation to sun, altitude or extreme weather conditions. Along with numerous other automatic functions these are all controlled from this most important centre of the Subconscious Brain.

The Hypothalamus has a rear chamber filled with brain fluid (CSF). Its roof has the analytical centres of emotions - rage, passion, happiness, fear, sorrow, jealousy, revenge and sexual pleasure which we feel them here and react through the Hypothalamus which expresses emotions via hormones. At the rear end of this chamber, we have the Pineal Gland which produces the hormone Melatonin, the night hormone responsible for rest and sleep.

Just below the Hypothalamus, and in front of it lies the highly protected Pituitary Gland. This gland rests in a chamber guarded on three sides by a part of the skull called the Saddle. This is where all the hormones are regulated and is the true headquarters of our hormonal system such as the thyroid, adrenals, ovaries, testes, melanin production (for pigmentation of the skin). The Hypothalamus and Pituitary work together as the former gives the commands which the latter executes. Our immune system; sense of well-being; energy; healing power; stress levels; ageing are all controlled by these two interlinked structures of the Subconscious Brain. This is often referred to as "The Hypothalamic-Pituitary Axis".

The third floor houses the Mid Brain (Mesencephalon). This part of the brain maintains consciousness, so keeps us awake and alert. Chronic fatigue and excessive sleep – like Narcolepsy – are related to this part of the brain.

The second level of the brain consists of the Pons (meaning 'bridge'). This is the link that connects the Midbrain with the Brain Stem and Cerebellum, which is the mini brain, lying beneath the main brain. The surfaces of these two 'brains' look similar but have completely different functions. The Cerebellum controls posture and fine tuning of gait; writing; acquired skills like playing a musical instrument, dancing, knitting and all the activities we do automatically without being seriously 'mindful'. Some scientists think it is the most intelligent part of the brain. It communicates with Nature and adapts to its changes.

The Pons has the nuclei or nerve centres, for the eye muscles, inner ear, facial muscles etc here also lies the centre that controls the rhythm of breathing. If something is not right here, the result is palpitations.

The lowest part of the brain consists of the stem of the brain called the Medulla Oblongata, as it is oblong–shaped. This connects the brain with the spinal cord that runs down the entire length of the back. The most important centre in this part is the one that controls both breathing and heartbeat. The forces with which these vital organs functions are automatically controlled from these two centres. There are many nerve centres here that control saliva secretion, facial expression, tongue movement, gum sensations, teeth, face, taste buds, hearing etc thus the Medulla Oblongata is also a very important part of the brain. Moreover, all the information passing to the various parts of the brain from the entire body and vice versa, pass through the nerve fibres located here.

I cannot stress enough the importance of the Subconscious Brain. Later on, I will explain how diseases and well-being are linked to this part of the brain in the vast majority of cases and in particular the influence on it of the neck.

# Chapter 3 - The Discovery

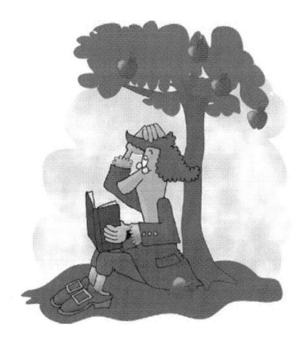

*When the apple fell on my head, I discovered that the subconscious brain has its own circulatory network known as the Vertebro-Basilar Network.*

This network forms an arterial circle around the Pituitary Gland (Circle of Willis, see figure Y). At this level additional blood is supplied to it from the arteries of the conscious brain as a back up (Internal Carotid Arteries). This is to ensure that Pituitary gland and the Hypothalamus get uninterrupted blood supply…

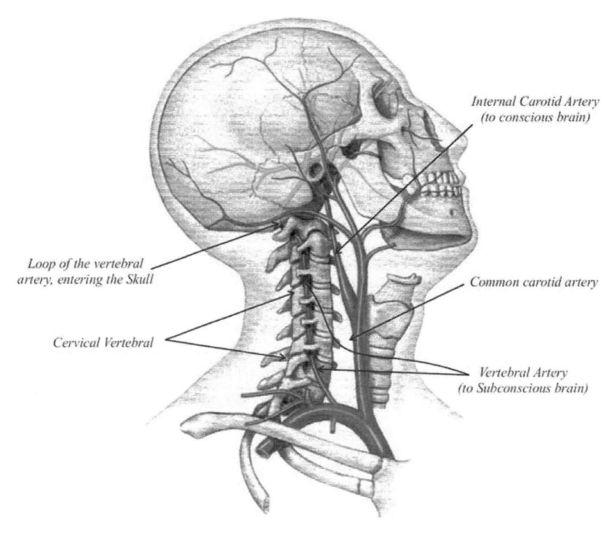

Internal Carotid Artery
(to conscious brain)

Loop of the vertebral
artery, entering the Skull

Cervical Vertebral

Common carotid artery

Vertebral Artery
(to Subconscious brain)

Figure (X)

(Branches of arteries emerging from the heart)

I began to study the anatomy of the neck. It has seven flat-bodied vertebrae, in a span of some 15 cm, whereas the entire back, which is normally over a metre long, has only 17 vertebrae. These flat vertebrae of the neck are light and flexible. Our sensory organs, such as our eyes, ears and nose are directional so our head has to turn frequently to see, hear and smell. The rest of the spine is less flexible. Here lies the problem. Since the neck is flexible, it is more prone to traumas and dislocation. Thus in terms of pain or stiffness, our neck gives us more trouble than any other part of the body.

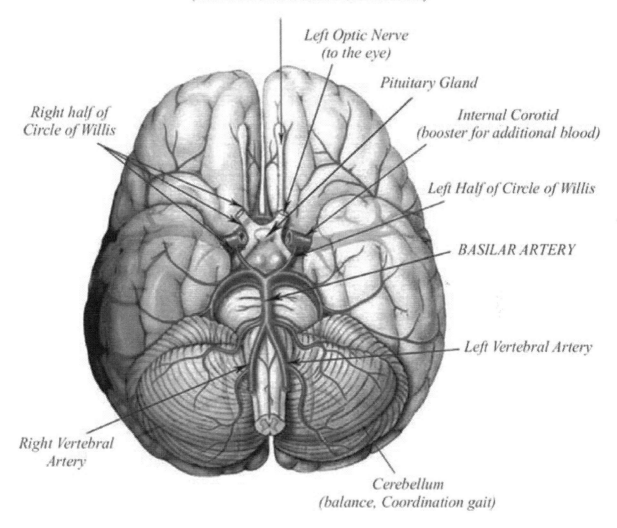

*(OLFACTORY BULB FOR SMELL)*

*Left Optic Nerve*
*(to the eye)*

*Pituitary Gland*

*Right half of*
*Circle of Willis*

*Internal Corotid*
*(booster for additional blood)*

*Left Half of Circle of Willis*

*BASILAR ARTERY*

*Left Vertebral Artery*

*Right Vertebral*
*Artery*

*Cerebellum*
*(balance, Coordination gait)*

Figure (Y)

(Blood vessels (arteries) on the inferior surface of the brain)

As I mentioned earlier, the vertebral arteries, our better 'life source', run through a pair of canals located in the first five vertebrae of the neck, inside their wings (see Figure X). Then they emerge; make a loop and join together to form the Basiler Artery at the base of the brain, which is located on the lower surface of the Medulla Oblongata. At this point, it is already inside the skull, so its protection is ensured. Neither the Axis nor Atlas has any room for the vertebral arteries, as they move excessively and so the risk of trauma to them is high. Here Nature has a shortcoming in that it has protected the vital Vertebral Arteries except for 2cms or so, when they come out of the canals and form the loop before entering the protected space of the skull. Thus, between the base of the Axis and the No. 3 vertebra of the neck, the arteries are covered not by bones but by a sheath of thick ligament. Unfortunately, ligaments are not bones and after head injuries, whiplash injuries, falls, traumas of labour etc, these can tear or get stretched. This results in the compression of the arteries, despite their strength and elasticity, whenever the neck muscles get stiff from stress, excessive computer use etc.

Many head and neck injuries caused by trauma result in dislocation of the facet joints of the cervical vertebrae. In my opinion, the most common are of the first four vertebrae. The dislocation causes misalignment of the cervical spine. The shifted vertebrae pull or twist the vertebral arteries. The blood flow through the Vertebral Arteries is then restricted or the flow becomes turbulent. This compression of the arteries ultimately causes a malfunction of the Subconscious Brain, often with disastrous consequences.

## Effect on the Brain

The brain cells are highly specialized and they need 'fuel' to function all the time. They do not have any reserve fat or carbohydrate storage facility. They instantly utilize what is available. Moreover, there exists a strict blood-brain barrier: not everything that is carried by blood can permeate into brain cells. This barrier facilitates the passage of safe products and chemicals to the brain, again ensuring that there is no damage done to the brain cells. Oxygen and glucose are easily accessible to the brain cells. In fact, the brain cells are highly susceptible to a decrease in the supply of oxygen and glucose levels. We know very well that when sugar levels in the blood or the brain, drop the effect is hypoglycaemia (hypo- less, glycogen or sugar) and is alarming, as the person experiences shivering, fainting sensation, a cold sweat, panic etc Lack of oxygen (as at high altitude) causes palpitations, tingling, an irregular breathing pattern, fainting etc

Alcohol, narcotic drugs, tranquillizers, tobacco, sedatives, certain chemotherapy drugs etc, cross the blood-brain barrier and reach the brain cells to produce their respective effect. Some drugs, especially those used recreationally such as Speed, Ecstasy etc, are chemically engineered to break this barrier. Alcohol's effect on the brain is traditionally so obvious. First, it relaxes the mind, and then excites it, before the drinker collapses into a comatose state, when the level of alcohol in the brain is high.

The oxygen and glucose supply to the brain are together the key controller of its function. We all know that if the oxygen supply to the brain is stopped for approximately four minutes, the brain cells change and can die. That is how sensitive they are. Other cells, like muscles and bone scan survive for several hours or days. If the blood supply to the toes is blocked, by diabetic or frostbite conditions, the necrosis or death of the cells, takes a while to develop. After a snake bite, it is common practice to tie the arm or thigh, very tightly with a rope so that the blood supply is totally cut-off, until help is received. This may take several hours and after anti-venom treatment is given, the compressed limb recovers its full function.

In suicide by hanging, death comes quickly. As the blood-flow to the brain is cut-off, the person goes to sleep and doesn't feel anything. Just before death, there is a sudden jerk and all voluntary and involuntary functions cease. At the very last minute, the person may involuntarily urinate or defecate as the corresponding sphincters dilate. The subconscious brain releases all that it controls.

These are dramatic situations. In the majority of cases, it is the malfunctioning of the brain tissue and the various centres of the Sub-conscious Brain which matters most. In my experience and with logical (non-scientific) analysis, I have found that if the blood flow to the Subconscious Brain is reduced by 40%, it begins to malfunction and chronic fatigue sets in. The person feels tired, lethargic, listless etc and most voluntary functions, such as walking, talking, thinking, making decisions, comprehension etc, slow down as well. If the blood flow is reduced further, by about 60%, the person experiences headaches, nausea, sickness, extreme fatigue, loss of muscle power, extreme sensitivity to light, dizziness, imbalance etc If the blood flow to the Subconscious Brain is reduced by 80%, then the person gets panic attacks, epileptic fits, tinnitus, sees flashing lights, palpitations and has tremors in the body etc If the blood to the Subconscious Brain is reduced by more than 80%, then fainting occurs and a person will collapse. All parts of the body shut-down and only the heart and lungs are kept active, because Nature tries to conserve oxygen for the functioning of these two vital organs. If the oxygen supply through blood stops totally for 4 minutes, the brain then suffers irreversible changes. Its proteins change and the cell walls loose their functions. If, on the other hand, the body is in a frozen state and the heart stops because of that, such as drowning in an ice-cold lake, then the cells of the heart and respiration centres are kept inert. The brain tissue in this state does not go through irreversible changes. This feature can be used in heart surgery. While I was a student in Moscow, we observed how open-heart surgery was performed by cooling the blood to 4 degrees Celsius. The requirement for oxygen in the brain decreases to a minimum in freezing conditions. Animals, such as bears, can hibernate for months during the cold winter months, while breathing only occasionally so that only life-sustaining functions can continue.

In the early 70's, a strange experiment was carried out by international scientists in Delhi. An expert of Yoga, known as a Yogi, was buried alive in a coffin and his heart was monitored by an ECG machine. His heart slowed down to about 10 beats per minute; enough to supply the basic amount of oxygen to the brain. He was in a hibernative state. He remained there for almost 7 days. When dug out, he was able to breathe and function normally. This yogi used his powers of the Conscious Brain and suppressed or slowed down the heart beat and breathing rate. His metabolism slowed down and he needed basic "fuel" (oxygen and glucose) to survive.

Decreased blood supply to the brain can diminish its functions. If there is anaemia or low blood pressure, the effect is obvious. The person feels very tired, has mild palpitations, yawns and sighs a lot, feels dizziness, has headaches and has a 'sinking feeling' in the heart. Again, after a heavy meal, the blood rushes to the stomach and intestines to aid digestion by churning the stomach to break-up food, increase gastric juice secretion, provide for movement of food through the intestines and absorption of digested food etc This deprives the brain of blood and so one feels very sleepy and often edgy if one has to work. This is why, in many countries, people take an afternoon siesta in order to avoid being under active after lunch.

Before menstruation, blood rushes to the lower abdomen to form a reserve in the pelvic region, in preparation for a sudden haemorrhage. This draws blood away from the brain, resulting in a range of physical and psychological symptoms known as Pre-menstrual Syndrome. About 3-7 days before the onset of the period, women may feel agitated, exhausted, emotional (often unreasonably), panicky, restless, suffer sleeplessness etc Water retention and painful breasts are hormone- related and they are caused by malfunctions of the Pituitary Gland caused by lack of adequate blood supply.

## The Role of CSF

Earlier, I mentioned Cerebro Spinal Fluid (CSF) in which the brain 'floats' (see Figure Z). This fluid penetrates various chambers and canal ways, located deep inside the brain. These are the backwaters of the sea of CSF which cover the outer surface of the brain. They are called ventricles. This fluid contains some oxygen, the level of which is the same as can be absorbed by water. However, the level of glucose in the CSF is substantial, so it can be an additional supply of fuel for both the inner and outer surfaces of the brain. It also contains some minerals which are dissolved in the liquid. The CSF cannot diffuse deep into the brain, so it is a secondary, but important, source of fuel for the brain.

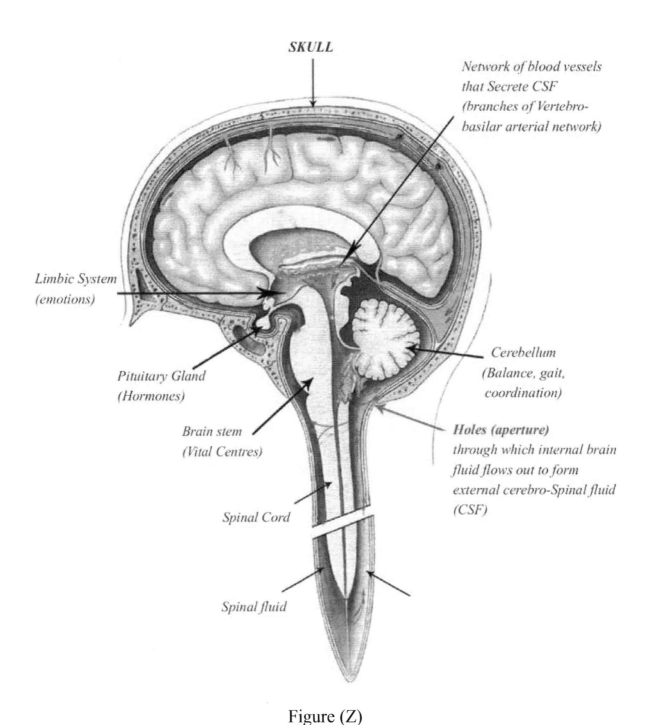

Figure (Z)

**(Formation and circulation of Cerebro-Spinal Fluid (CSF) or brain fluid)**

If there is a leakage of this CSF after an epidural injection in the lower back – in the case of anaesthesia for painless labour or pelvic surgery – the patient will suffer headaches, extreme fatigue and dizziness.

If excess fluid accumulates as in hydrocephaly (a large head, swollen with fluid) in babies, the brain surfaces are squashed due to the hydraulic pressure and the result is poor development of mental and physical capabilities and the child is often retarded.

Blood flow to the brain is more vital than CSF circulation because of the former's oxygen supplying capabilities, through its Red Blood Cells. Cranial Osteopaths generally help to improve the CSF circulation to the brain by gentle manipulation. My technique, which I call the 'Ali Technique', helps to improve both the blood and the CSF to the brain. The results from this technique are better and long-lasting.

## Restriction of Blood Supply to the Brain

In order to understand how important a constant and ample supply of blood to the brain is, we must look at the negative side. This is a purely logical approach. What happens to the body and its functioning when there is a reduced supply of blood to the brain? If you look at the extreme case of a stroke, when a blood clot forms in the heart due to an irregular heart beat, it travels along an artery and plugs one of the smaller blood vessels, the corresponding area of the brain is instantly starved of oxygen and glucose. That part of the brain soon dies. If the clot travels through the carotid artery to the cortical or conscious brain, there will be instant loss of muscle power on one side of the body and the person may even become unconscious. If the clot travels to the left half of the brain, where the speech centre is located in a right-handed person, there is a loss of speech. For that to happen to a left-handed person, the clot must travel to the right side of the brain. This is so because the nerve fibres from the brain cells cross over in the brain stem area to connect to the opposite side of the body. One half of the body is paralysed after a stroke.

If the clot travels up the Vertebral Arteries, the Subconscious Brain is starved of oxygen instantly. Depending on where the clot gets stuck, the corresponding part of the brain dies. If blood flow to the brain stem is blocked, then there is instant death, as both the heart and respiratory centres of the brain stop functioning. A clot along the Vertebral Artery is usually fatal, which is again a proof that the Subconscious Brain is vital to our existence and the arteries that feed it are the most important blood vessels, besides the coronary (or heart) arteries, in the entire body.

## Causes of narrowing of the canal in the neck

The following are some of the causes of narrowing of the canal in the neck, gathered by me over 20 years of practice:

1.  **Misalignment of the neck vertebrae** due to whiplash injuries, birth injuries like forceps or Ventouse delivery; head and neck injuries; boxing; tumbling, as in a skiing accident; falls from heights or horseback; walking into glass doors; hitting the head on a beam when walking; excessive dental work; long anaesthesia during surgery (when the head is pushed back and there is no resistance); cutting the jaw; breaking the nose; an embryo lying with the face squashed in the uterus especially with twins; being dropped as a child or falling from a cot; tumbling downstairs; motor cycle accidents; brawls or domestic violence; habitually sleeping on the stomach for many years; lying with the head twisted in rubble after an earthquake; frequent bungee jumping etc

2.  **Compression of the disks** of the vertebrae of the neck, resulting in narrowing or kinks, in the vertebral arteries. Causes include doing yogic headstands without preparation; objects falling on the head; head-on collisions in Rugby; hitting the head on taxi or car doors; falling head down; diving into the wall of a swimming pool; very rapid labour through a tight birth canal ('Champagne cork' birth within 30 minutes to 1 hour); severe contraction during labour with the opening of the birth canal tightly closed, labour in the breech position with strong contraction on the head of the baby; motor car accident, when it overturns and lies upside down; a tree falling on the head; earthquake with trauma to the head when the ceiling collapses; rod or stick hitting in fights; accident of stuntmen when objects hit the head; a rod falling on the head whilst weight-lifting,

prolonged labour in breach position when uterine muscles press the head, hitting a beam with the head etc

3.  **Sudden lateral movement of the head and neck** due to falling-off a horse; skiing accidents; football injuries, punches on the cheeks as in boxing or fights; martial arts injuries to the side of the face from kicking sideways; car being hit from the side; spinning in a car accident; facial surgeries under anaesthesia; difficult extraction of molar or premolar tooth (on the side of the mouth), trampoline accidents, trauma after a bomb explosion etc

4.  **Repetitive movements of the head and neck** as in dancing; frequent use of the telephone with the head tilted to one side; sports injuries (Rugby, American football), wrestling injuries, frequent flights etc

5.  **Poor mobility as a result of calcium deposits** on the facet joints of the cervical vertebrae; working posture; narrowing of the spinal canal (where the spinal cord is located) due to disc protruding in the spinal canal causing pain and stiffness of the neck; crushing of the neck vertebrae from old fractures etc

6.  **Neck stiffness due to poor mobility** caused by excessive computer use (typically more than 6 hours a day), driving, knitting, sedentary desk jobs, playing the violin with the neck held in the same position for a long time, lying in bed for many days (typically due to fractures of the spinal bones), using neck collars for many days etc Arab men who wear head gears (not turbans) have to fix their head up right as the round band they wear is likely to slip. They are very conscious of that embarrassing situation. Strong wind awkward movements, running, bending down can make the head gear slip. They have a lot of neck pain due to this.

7.  **Neck stiffness due to imposed conditions** such as Osteoporosis, when the neck shrinks; Ankylosis or fusion of the joints of the cervical spine due to an auto-immune disease; putting titanium discs in the spine; fixing a rod (Harrington's) in the neck to immobilize it in extreme neck damage or degenerative scoliosis, arthritis of the joints

of the neck; paraplegia (paralysis from the neck down after a spinal injury) etc

8. **If plaque (Atherosclerosis) is formed** in the inner lining of vertebral arteries due to high cholesterol, smoking, diabetes, ageing etc the reduction of blood flow is permanent. People have frequent "Mini stroke (TIA)", faint, vertigo, Tinnitus as in old age because of this.

These conditions severely affect the neck, whose shape and functioning is modified. Blood flow to the brain is then simultaneously reduced.

There are other causes which affect the general blood circulation and deprive the brain. These may be temporary or long-term. After a heavy meal the blood forms a depot around the stomach area. This reduces the total amount of blood reaching the brain. Thus, one feels drowsy or lethargic after a meal. Before menstruation begins there is a tendency to pelvic congestion. The blood forms a depot around the uterus, in case there is a severe haemorrhaging during the period. Acute blood-loss due to blood-letting, trauma or surgery, blood donation, severe dehydration, leeching, anaemia, very low blood pressure, arrhythmic heartbeat (missing beats), atrial fibrillation- when the heart 'flutters' etc, all reduce the amount of oxygen to the brain. Those teenagers, who grow very quickly, which are quite a common phenomenon nowadays, can have very long necks. If they also suffer from low blood pressure the brain will get less blood and it will function poorly. Such teenagers are often tired and irritable, suffering from lack of concentration, poor immune system, excessive acne, cravings for sweets or chocolates, insomnia etc. In aerobatics, negative G-force can cause blackout for a brief period. They see pink when they have positive G-force while flying and see grey or blackout with negative G-force.

Imagine you are watering the garden. Some areas get more water than others. That depends on the uneven surface density of the grass, distance from the source etc if the pressure of the water in the hose pipe is low and not enough flows through it, those areas will receive very little water; some areas will only receive a trickle. Similar things happen in the brain. There are numerous blood vessels and they are not perfect in shape and size (rather like our face, eyes nose, thumb prints etc). Even when the pressure or volume, of blood running through it is adequate, the various parts of the brain get varying amounts of blood.

The chances of obstruction to the smooth flow of blood through this pair of arteries are very high. This is the price we Homo sapiens have to face for walking erect. Our predecessors, the four-legged animals, moved horizontally and so the blood from the heart went straight through the canals to the brain. The pressure was adequate to overcome any mild compression. However, when a dog sits too long on its hind legs begging it sometimes goes to sleep and falls over. Humans face the same problem by walking vertically. We have to pump blood against gravity so even the slightest resistance along the path of the canals can result in poor irrigation of the brain. Giraffes, when swinging their head, are often disorientated (they probably feel dizzy) because of their long neck. Reaching for green leaves on the top of the tree has been made easy, but eating grass and then moving the head up can cause discomfort.

The key issue is that different parts of the Subconscious Brain have different functions. The symptoms that arise from malfunction of various nerve or control centres or of major functions of the body can vary. Some may be psychological in nature, while others could be physical (palpitation, extreme fatigue, headaches, imbalance etc) but the cause is the same: reduced blood supply.

These symptoms will be discussed in the next chapter under the heading 'The Ali Syndrome', which is how it became known in my clinic.

## Stress

We conclude this chapter by talking about the role stress plays in increasing the demand of oxygen in the brain and simultaneously cutting-off the supply chain. It is a bizarre reaction. In stress, it is obvious that the brain cells will be hyperactive and so they need more blood. This high demand brings in more fluid to the brain (CSF) because it too has glucose and some oxygen. As the fluid accumulates in the brain canals, cisterns and the skull, the pressure on the brain surface increases. This tightens the neck very quickly to stop more fluid formation. This tightening of the neck muscles causes reduction of blood flow through vertebral arteries. The subconscious brain then gets less blood.

In Meningitis, there is increased fluid pressure in the brain and thus the first symptom is tightness of the neck muscles. The Dutch name for Meningitis is 'Nek Kramp' (neck cramp). When a child cries, the neck becomes very tight with stress. Barking dogs are stressed and their neck muscles also tighten-up.

The neck muscles are attached to the occiput or back of the skull. Stress, excessive computer use long durations etc causes tightening of these muscles. The head is slightly pulled back. This compresses the vertebral arteries where they form the loop (see Figure A) and seriously impair blood flow.

There is a short-term or acute stress, like a burst of anger. When the situation calms down the neck muscles relax. Chronic conditions, however, stress the body and tighten the neck permanently in anticipation. Stress, therefore, can cause prolonged reduction of blood flow to the subconscious brain. That, in my opinion, is the logical explanation of why stress is linked to so many diseases. The failure of a particular brain centre leads to the breaking down of functions of the corresponding organs or systems. Weakening of the immune system is direct result of stress.

I have not found any mention in Medicine where scientists have been able to explain why prolonged stress causes us so much harm. I sincerely hope that sceptics will accept my hypothesis and carry out experiments to prove or disprove it.

# Chapter 4 - The Ali Syndrome

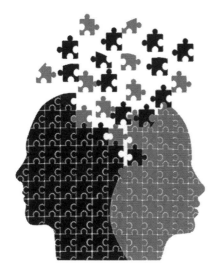

*The Ali Syndrome is not a disease, even though we know it results from poor blood supply to the subconscious brain, from whatever cause.*

First of all, what is a syndrome? One could say a causeless condition.

A disease is characterised by the presence of a cause. Thus, bronchitis, viral meningitis, bacteria dysentery, arthritis, cystitis etc, are called diseases. We can pin point the cause like inflammation (a suffix 'itis' means inflammation), a virus, bacteria etc.

A syndrome is not a disease as it is difficult to point out the 'cause' of this condition. In reality, a Syndrome is a collection of symptoms which mayor may not, be linked. There is usually no single cause that manifests as symptoms. Here are some examples:

a) Down's Syndrome: The cause is an extra 21$^{st}$ pair of chromosomes. There are three instead of two prints of the chromosome. The syndrome is characterised by 'mongoloid' (slit eyes, round face) face, mental retardation, and defects in the cardiovascular system.

b) Polycystic Ovarian Syndrome (PCOS): This is characterised by multiple cysts in the ovary. This syndrome comprises dysfunction of periods, weight gain, facial hair, insulin-resistance (which could lead to diabetes) and acne.

c) Irritable Bowel Syndrome (IBS): This is characterised by frequent diarrhoea, bloating, abdominal cramps, occasional constipation, indigestion, flatulence etc the actual cause of such varying symptoms is not known, but they are often present in a batch.

## About The Ali Syndrome

The Ali Syndrome is not a disease, even though we know it results from poor blood supply to the subconscious brain, from whatever cause. The symptoms vary in intensity and may appear in various permutations and combinations according to the area of the subconscious brain most affected. I will discuss the symptoms according to their locations in the brain.

## The Limbic System (Emotional Centre)

(Limbus – border between the conscious and subconscious brain).

Symptoms include:

- Loss of drives: loss of libido, desire to do things and motivation.

- Loss of short-term memory, also storage and retrieval of memory.

- Loss of smell, taste

- Difficulty in swallowing

- Emotional disturbances, such as mood swings, depression, panic attacks, anxiety, becoming angry over small trivial things.

## The Pineal Gland

This gland, located at the rear end of the Hypothalamus area, secretes Melatonin, a hormone that is only produced at night. It is the main regulator of sleep. If Cortisol (Adrenaline) helps you to carryout your daytime activities, such as working, digestion, even just staying awake, then Melatonin helps you in rest and repose. The repair work of the wear and tear of the body, synthesis of blood cells, healing of cuts, bruises, traumas, replenishing the body's energy, removal of waste from the tissues, helping the liver to replenish energy are all carried out at night when the body is asleep. Thus, Melatonin is as vital as Cortisol, the main daytime hormone.

The blood vessels carry Melatonin secretion to the rest of the body. Malfunction, caused primarily by the failure of the vertebra basilar arterial network, can therefore have serious consequences.

Symptoms of poor Melatonin Secretion:

- Day-Night Circadian cycle is reversed. You are awake and 'buzzing' with thoughts at night and very tired and lethargic during the day. In other words, you have permanent Jet lag. Medicine has called it Insomnia, but if you look at it carefully, it is the alteration of the day and night cycle. True Insomnia or lack of sleep, is when you don't sleep at all, day or night as seen in many mental illness and extreme stress.

- Melatonin also helps the maturation of sperm and eggs; a function which is very delicate and requires a lot of energy. That energy is almost celestial. Sperm and egg production and release is a night time activity.

Some years ago, it was very fashionable to take synthetic Melatonin. It was thought to be a wonder drug. It may have helped some people to get slightly better sleep, but it didn't do much else. The message from the retina of the eye confirms that it's dark outside and the Pineal Gland begins to secrete Melatonin. The repair and replenishing of the body's energy is flagged up. If someone puts the light on in the room, the Melatonin production and secretion stops instantly. The person is then wide-awake and finds himself in difficulty, as going back to sleep will take some time. Thus light or darkness, determines its secretion.

Thus, sleep is essential for reproductive functions. Natural sleep is better than that induced by drugs.

## Hypothalamus and Pituitary

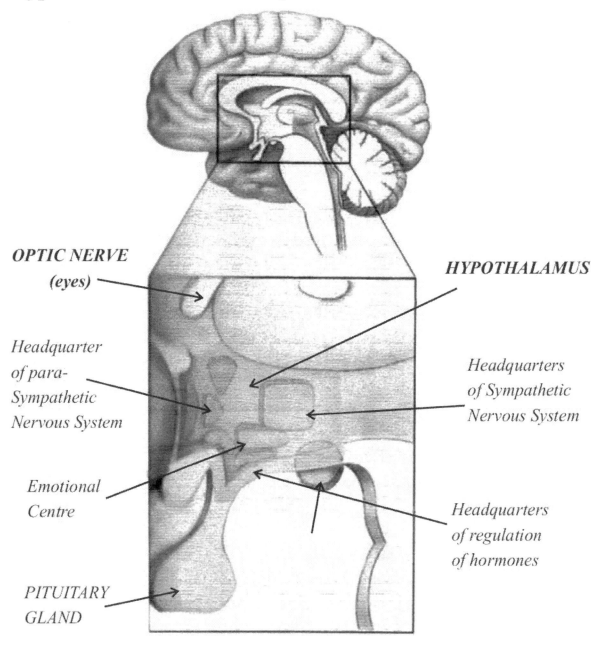

OPTIC NERVE
(eyes)

HYPOTHALAMUS

Headquarter
of para-
Sympathetic
Nervous System

Headquarters
of Sympathetic
Nervous System

Emotional
Centre

Headquarters
of regulation
of hormones

PITUITARY
GLAND

(section of the brain showing location of pituitary gland, hypothalamus, emotional centre)

## Hypothalamus

The Hypothalamus instructs the Pituitary to secrete specific hormones. Thus, they work together where the Hypothalamus analyzes the situation in the body or mind and then commands the Pituitary to secrete the right or predicted amount of the given hormone.

For example, if you are in a stressful situation and you need to react immediately, here is how the chain reaction starts: the eyes send a message to the conscious brain, which instructs the Hypothalamus to respond. It analyses the information and makes an instantaneous decision for a response strategy. It commands the Pituitary to stimulate the adrenal glands (located above the kidneys) with a stimulating hormone (called ACTH). The adrenal glands then secrete Adrenaline or Cortisol, which is transported via blood to the heart, lungs, muscles, sweat glands etc The heart beats faster, the breathing rate increases, muscles tighten, the metabolic rate in muscles increases to produce more energy, sweating increases to 'cool' the body etc Nature has created hormones to do multi-tasking with minimum loss of time and energy.

The Hypothalamus is thus the main 'Intelligence' of the body. In the universe or nature too, there must be a 'Hypothalamus', which controls the solar system, the weather, seasons, and climate change as a response to human activities on earth

The interesting thing is that we can exercise some control over that autonomic world with some training of the conscious brain.

I have walked over hot marble in the Taj Mahal at midday; held my breath for 1 minute 30 seconds; turned my hand hot or cold at will; elongated my fingers by over a centimetre at will; slowed down my heart rate by 20%, slept without a blanket at a temperature of below 20 degrees C. I am not boasting, but meditation and breath control, over a period of a number of years, can help anyone do this. There are people who have gone even further. I know of a person who did 'Samadhi', a higher yogic method of stopping heart and breathing activity altogether to slip into a hibernation and finally death. It's hard to believe this, but it does happen in India and in Buddhist practices. Thus the conscious brain can be trained to influence the Hypothalamus, the headquarters of the subconscious brain.

There are numerous caves in Tibet where mummified bodies of such monks are still to be found. In Gui, in the Spiti Valley in the Indian Himalayas, where I often trek, there is one such mummified monk in a small temple. The mummy is over 500 years old and is totally intact. No one, however, has done any internal examination. There are several caves in the Tabo villages where Buddhist monks went into Samadhi (a higher level of concentrated meditation) after completion of their worldly mission in their current life. They sat in the Lotus position, controlled breath, and heart rate, cut off from feeling the environment, remained in trance and stepped into Samadhi. Call it euthanasia or a spiritual journey; it's your choice.

The main parameters of the life force, the Immune System, Adaptation and Homeostasis, are entirely controlled and managed by the Hypothalamus-Pituitary complex as follows:

## 1. The Immune System

This protects us from harm by neutralizing or destroying, invading bodies. If this is a living bacterium or virus, the body's immune system produces antibodies to neutralize it

If the particles are non-living: pollen, seeds or nuts, pollutants, gluten in wheat, egg protein, dog or cat hair etc, the body's reaction is through the allergy response. The Hypothalamus identifies these allergens after receiving information from lymphocytes (white blood cells in the blood) and initiates a chemical-hormonal response to the situation. The hormone released by the Basophils (another type of white blood cells) is Histamine.

By the way, an allergic reaction produced by histamines in the body is a good thing. That is to say that the immune system is functioning well, but unfortunately, the actual reaction can be very unpleasant. Runny nose, sneezing, asthma, itchy eyes and skin, unpleasant-looking rashes on the body etc, are major irritants. We take anti-histamines to block the histamine so that it cannot produce such annoying symptoms. In an ideal world we should use natural methods of desensitization so that the body does not respond so violently and becomes more tolerant.

Sometimes the body's own tissues, like joint surfaces, skin, eyes, gut, kidneys etc, become the target for the immune system. The Hypothalamus receives a message saying that some traitors have 'changed their loyalty to the body'. The angry immune system goes out in full force to destroy these cells, causing a very undesirable reaction called 'Autoimmune Disease'. The body tries to destroy its own tissue because of some misinterpretation. These diseases are Rheumatoid Arthritis, Lupus, Psoriasis, Vitiligo (white patches), Crohn's Disease, Ulcerative Colitis, Nephritis (kidney disease) Scleroderma (when the skin hardens and acquires a leather-like texture), Ulcerative Colitis, Hashimoto's Thyroid Disease etc

These conditions are difficult to treat, as we still do not know why these tissues become denatured. The hypothalamus or the immune system is doing its job well, even though serious suffering may result. Steroids and strong immunosuppressants are used to symptomatically treat these conditions. I have some solutions to this problem and they will be discussed later.

The Immune System is an extended function of the Innate Healing Power. Its main role is to protect us from foreign bodies or particles, from settling down in the body. Imagine the opposite, as in the case of AIDS (Acquired Immuno Deficiency Syndrome), where the Immune System functions poorly. All sorts of viral, bacterial and fungal infections (for example from using too many antibiotics for bacterial infections) slowly destroy the body. It results in death.

The Hypothalamus-Pituitary axis can function poorly when it is irrigated insufficiently. Cranial Osteopaths have long established that children born with forceps or Ventouse delivery and those with head and neck injuries at birth or later develop eczema, asthma and are generally very 'chesty', with frequent colds and coughs. Their immune system is poor. Gentle Cranio-Sacral work establishes good flow of the CSF and the Hypothalamus-Pituitary also gets additional nutrition. This cures such problems.

A clinical trial carried out in a leading London Hospital showed that Cranial Osteopathy helped to change immunological markers in blood for the better.

My techniques, which are more to do with blood than CSF circulation in the brain, showed remarkable results. In 1994, I gathered case histories of some twenty-five children and went to meet Dr Andrew Bush at the Royal Brompton Hospital in London, UK. He was a consultant in Respiratory Disease. I explained my technique of diet, neck massage and yogic breathing exercise for the treatment of Asthma. He was very impressed, but the Research Committee found the approach too anecdotal and opted for a different trial using complementary medicine. 'Where is the catch?' they asked, too many therapies were applied simultaneously.

Later in this book I will discuss another case where, years later, Professor Andrew Bush was completely taken aback by a beautiful 3 year old Russian girl having her life saved by these techniques.

## 2. Adaptation

This is a unique phenomenon in all living beings. The Hypothalamus assesses the changes in the environment and brings about physiological and emotional adjustments so that the body and the mind can cope with the situation.

If you go to a hot and sunny place, fair skin acquires a tan within hours. The bright sun can damage the skin and the pigment melanin helps to block it.

If you go to an altitude, the lack of oxygen makes you breathe differently until such time when the bone marrow produces more haemoglobin and Red Blood Cells. If you are at 2,000 metres, a healthy body may take two days to adjust. If you go above 3,000 metres, you may need five days to adapt.

I have led treks in the higher Himalayas over the past twenty years. In the beginning, we experienced a lot of complications, such as pounding headaches, altered breathing – faster and faster at first and then at the peak breathing stops for a few seconds and then start all over again. This is called Cheyne-Stokes breathing. In Sleep Apnoea, a condition that sounds very scary to a companion, a similar breathing pattern is noticed. Those who go into a coma have similar breathing, but nowadays ventilators change the breathing artificially.

One year, I took to the trek my therapists, who gave us all an hour's massage. It took much less time to adapt as my technique was applied to improve the blood flow to the brain. Now we have made it a standard feature for each group, so nausea, panic attacks and fainting are a thing of the past.

### 3.  Homeostasis (homeo – unchanging; statis –standing)

This is a phenomenon in the body that maintains harmony. The pH of the blood is a constant 7.4. You may drink a litre of lemon juice, but the blood will be automatically alkalised so that the pH value remains the same. The cells function optimally at that pH level (7 is normal and 7.4 is slightly alkaline).

The level of blood cells, sugar, protein, salts, cholesterol, uric acid, body temperature, heart rate, breathing rate, day-night cycle etc are all kept in harmony within certain ranges. Nature knows that cells function optimally in a certain environment, so it works around the clock to maintain that balance or harmony through the Hypothalamus-Pituitary system.

If, for example, some bacteria or viruses enter the body, in a defensive tactic the thermostat in the hypothalamus is adjusted to raise the body temperature so that the invading organisms cannot thrive. They too like a cosy environment. The use of Paracetamol, however, confuses the temperature regulatory system (thermostat), which suddenly notices that the body temperature is too high so it instructs the sweat glands to open and secrete. The sweat evaporates on the skin and the body temperature or fever, falls to its near-normal level. This is an example of sacrificing the natural cure for the sake of comfort.

Homeostasis is absolutely essential for our survival. This is the pillar that supports the Innate Healing Power. The disease processor pathogenic force, overcomes the health processor sanogenic forces, to cause an illness. Homeostasis, an arm of the Innate Healing Power, re-harmonises the body's chemistry and immune system, to bring them back to the optimum level in order to create health. The Hypothalamus-Pituitary Axis controls homeostasis.

# Functions of the Pituitary Gland

The Pituitary Gland secretes hormones that control the functions of vital organs and systems; the thyroid gland, the adrenal glands, the reproductive glands, blood sugar regulation, growth, water regulation, labour, pigmentation on the skin, immune system etc

## 1. The Thyroid Gland (controller of Metabolism)

This is the body's main regulator of metabolism (total chemical processes). Its hormone, Thyroxine, production is stimulated by the Pituitary, via the hormone, appropriately called the Thyroid Stimulating Hormone (TSH). Lack of Thyroxine production is commonly called 'low thyroid', which is known as Hypothyroidism (Hypo- low). When that has occurred, the metabolic rate (the 'burning' of fuel in the cells to produce energy) slows down. There is cellulite or white fat accumulation on the body, swelling of the body, intolerance to heat, period disturbances, slow motivation, which makes you lazy, with dry skin, low body temperature, hair loss, menstrual problems, chronic fatigue, depression, body aches etc It is as if there is a 'power failure' in the body and nothing works.

As iodine is an essential element in the production of Thyroxine, any such deficiency in the diet often leads to Hypothyroidism. Those who believe in Natural Medicine, therefore, take Sea Kelp, which is rich in Iodine to help Hypothyroidism.

Sometimes the opposite happens and the thyroid gland produces excess Thyroxine. That causes an increase in the metabolic rate. The skin is flushed, it is moist with sweat, the heart rate increases often causing irregular beats, the blood pressure increases as a result, there is anxiety, tremor in the hands' many suffer diarrhoea, weight loss, insomnia etc In spite of high excitation in the body, the person feels shattered and cannot function. This condition is called 'overactive thyroid' or Hyperthyroidism. In this case the Pituitary may not be the main cause. There is often a tumour in the thyroid gland called 'goitre' with hyperactive cells producing excess Thyroxine.

## 2. The Adrenal Glands

These are a yellow pyramid-shaped pair of gland that sits on the kidneys. They are only 7.5 grams in weight, but their action on the body is powerful. The yellow colour is due to the presence of stored lipids or fat molecules, like cholesterol and fatty acids, the raw material for production of the adrenal hormones in the adrenal gland. These hormones are collectively known as corticosteroids (these are 'steroids' found naturally in the body). So vital are these corticosteroids for the body that if the glands are removed, the body will die unless they are replaced by artificial steroids (the very hormones we are all conscious of).

Use of artificial steroids confuses the Hypothalamus and it begins to think that the adrenal cortex is functioning well, so it stops further stimulation. The cells of the adrenal cortex become lazy and can atrophy from lack of stimulation. This amounts to the total loss of functions of the adrenal cortex and one needs to be artificially stimulated. Steroids are 'emergency' hormones and should not be circulating in the blood all the time. Artificial steroids have many side effects like osteoporosis, weakening of the defences of the immune system, damage to the liver and kidneys, swellings on the body (especially the face) etc Thus, steroids should be administered with extreme caution.

The adrenal glands also secrete androgens or male hormones, similar to testosterone. If it is overactive in women they may develop muscles, grow a beard, lose hair on the scalp, deposit cellulite on the arms and thighs, have large breasts etc especially if the ovaries have cysts and fail to convert androgens into oestrogen.

Excess androgen (DHEA, male hormones) is unwanted in a female body. It is converted or aromatized by fat cells into a female hormone ESTROGEN, which is deposited as cellulite (white non-dietary, soft, with a cottage-cheese texture) in specific areas. These areas lie below the belly-button to resemble early pregnancy; something most women hate, around the waist, from the hip down to the knee on the thighs, from the shoulder to the elbow and in the breast. The cellulite spares the face and other parts of the body.

This esterone can also be produced in men due to a crisis of mistaken identity; In this case men develop breasts and have the body shape of a woman with cellulite (fat thighs, lower belly, fat arms etc). Many teenagers suffer from this condition in puberty. These boys get such a complex as peers tease them about their breasts. They stop swimming, lock doors when changing clothes, shun T-shirts that may divulge their breasts etc

Prolonged stress in women leads to hyper stimulation of the adrenal cortex by the hypothalamus-pituitary, leading to the cellulite deposits. These women control their diet, eat sparingly and try their best to avoid fats and sugar, but the weight just keeps increasing. I have written about this type of weight gain (Hormonal Weight Gain) in my book 'Dr Ali's Weight loss Plan' and 'Dr Ali's Woman's Health Bible'.

The innermost part of the adrenal gland secretes adrenaline. There is always some amount of these hormones secreted in the blood to keep us going, if there is an emergency or stressful situation and the body needs a heightened response, the hypothalamus stimulates this part, via the sympathetic nervous system. Large amounts of adrenaline are secreted in the blood. Stored glucose in the liver and muscles is released to produce extra energy. The heart rate, breathing rate, tension in the muscles and the metabolic rate increase to create the classic 'fight' or flight' reaction.

When a fox sees a rabbit, its adrenaline prepares it for a fight or chase, whilst the rabbit in fear also under the influence of the same hormone, is ready for flight. The emotions are different, but the body's reaction is the same.

If a stressful situation continues for days or months, the adrenaline secretion is constant. The body is in a permanent state of alertness and anxiety, as if it is fighting a running battle. This exhausts the body and there is an ultimate breakdown of the hypothalamic control system. This manifests into short or long-term illness like high blood pressure, auto-immune disease, psychological conditions, IBS, cancer etc.

## 3. The Reproductive system

The main Pituitary hormones, that stimulate testicular tissue in males and ovarian tissue in females, are FSH (Follicle Stimulating Hormone) and LH (Luteinising Hormone). These increase the production of Testosterone in males and Estrogen in women.

In females, these hormones first mature the 'follicles' or cells that contain egg cells. The most matured follicle releases a single egg and 'ovulation' takes place. The empty follicle then begins to secrete progesterone, which prepares the uterine lining to receive a potentially fertilized egg. The lining of the uterus thickens and if the egg is not fertilised within their 4-5 day lifespan, then the progesterone prepares to break up the uterine lining and the period starts. Thus, the menstrual cycle and fertility of women are controlled by the Hypothalamus-Pituitary axis.

## 4. Blood Sugar Regulation

The Pancreas has a dual function. It secretes pancreatic juice that digests protein, fats and carbohydrates in the intestines. The other function is that it regulates blood sugar, by means of insulin and glucagon secretion in the blood. While insulin uses-up excess glucose by sweeping it off into the cells, glucagon releases more glucose by breaking-down stored chemicals in the liver and muscles. These two hormones have contradicting functions and yet the cells that produce them are neighbours.

Again, this is a perfect example of homeostatis or the self-regulatory phenomenon that maintains harmony and equilibrium in the body. The Hypothalamus has an indirect or direct, role in maintaining the balance. When the system breaks-up, as in Diabetes, the insulin production is either inadequate or the cells of the body are too damaged to allow insulin to prepare them to accept glucose. When insulin is insufficient, because the pancreatic cells don't produce it, Type I or Insulin Dependent Diabetes sets in. If the glucose utilization by cells is poor, even though enough insulin is produced, then the result is excess blood sugar and this is called Type II Diabetes.

In this case the cell-walls are either damaged by free-radicals or overworked due to excessive consumption of sugar and alcohol.

### 4. Growth

Although the Pituitary secretes the Growth Hormone until around twenty-one years of age, other hormones such as Insulin, Thyroxin, and Cortisol from the adrenals, reproductive hormones like Testosterone and Oestrogen, especially during puberty, also help growth and repair of cells. Pituitary Growth Hormone helps the skeletal system to grow. Many adults who are short in height have a history of birth or other head and neck injury before puberty. This has been my analysis over the years.

Excess Growth Hormone can boost height at puberty. Many teenagers suffer from growing pains. The bone shafts and spine grow rapidly and the attached muscles cannot cope. This results in, often, excruciating pain in muscle tendons in the groin, knees, Achilles tendon etc

Hormones can affect moods. Those who take steroids know how agitated they feel. They cannot relax or sleep very well. At puberty, the surge of reproductive hormones makes teenagers very hyperactive, aggressive, unreasonable, hyper energetic etc

Hormones can contribute to premature ageing. The levels of Thyroid, water regulatory hormones, steroids, adrenalines etc remain unchanged with age. The insulin production may decrease, however, and this results in the elderly getting late-onset Diabetes. The Growth Hormone levels decrease and so repair work, muscle and bone building capacity drop. Thus, the elderly are more likely to develop muscle atrophy and osteoporosis.

Finally, the importance of the Hypothalamus- Pituitary- axis is demonstrated by the anatomy of the blood vessels. The two vertebral arteries join at the base of the brain to form a single Basilar Artery (Base artery). This artery bifurcates above the Pons and circles around the Pituitary. This ring of blood vessels, called the Circle of Willis, gets some additional blood from the Internal Carotid which is another artery that mostly feeds the conscious brain. Having lost blood to its various branches in the subconscious brain, its level drops and it gets some fresh supply from a neighbour (internal Carotid), so that the Hypothalamus-Pituitary gets ample blood. This boost in blood supply indicates that this area of the brain needs maximum and constant supply. The manufacture of hormones and coordinating functions of the body require extra energy. This is, after all, the Headquarters of the body's autonomous nervous system, our self-healing, self-regulatory, subconscious centers.

Another clever invention of Nature is that the Pituitary and other glands secrete their hormones into the venous system. This way they bypass the minute capillaries which lie at the end of the arteries. The veins carry the hormones quickly to the heart and then to the rest of the body. Thus the Vertebral Veins, located in the vertebral canals, are just as important as their accompanying arteries. They carry important hormones to the heart. Thus, obstruction to the blood-flow through these veins in the vertebral canal or the neck area has a serious effect on our health. They carry messenger hormones from the Pituitary to the target hormonal glands.

## Malfunction of the Pons

This part of the brain houses the nuclei or nerve centres, of several important cranial nerves. Lack of blood supply to the roots of these nerves, through tiny blood vessels called vasa nervorum (vas – vessels) or to the Pons directly, can cause:

- Bells' Palsy when one side of the face is paralysed, the eyes are wide open, the angle of the mouth drops.

- Lack of coordination of the eye muscles and sometimes double-vision.

- Tinnitus when the auditory nerve or its centre in the Pons does not get enough blood.

- Irregular breathing as in high altitude, panic attacks, coma etc

- Trigeminal neuralgia which is a serious painful disease affecting one half of the face or jaw or forehead. The Trigeminal Nerve has 3 branches (tri-three).

# Malfunction of the Cerebellum

There is a pair of arteries on each side of the Cerebellum that branch off the vertebral-basilar arteries. It is therefore well nourished. Although the function of the Cerebellum is not wholly understood, there is evidence that it is the main centre of coordination. We know that gait, posture, and balance are controlled from here. Besides these, perhaps other forms of coordination like playing music, singing, speaking, writing, driving, riding a bicycle etc must also be coordinated from here.

I have seen several patients who have had a stroke of the cerebellum. Their balance was severely affected and they suffered dizziness.

Increasingly excessive stress, computer use, trauma etc, neck injury or the tightness of muscles, impair blood flow to the cerebellum. Dizziness and nausea are therefore becoming more common. Even vertigo is becoming a recognisable medical condition. Most doctors blame the inner ear for it and often call it 'Meniere's Disease'. I have, however, successfully treated it with my technique, which should prove the cerebellum's blood supply was the culprit. A classic Meniere's disease is dizziness accompanied by tinnitus. I hope some doctors will read this and revise their opinion. I would, of course, understand the diagnosis if there were a problem with a tumour in the inner ear or some structural fault after injury. Sometimes, 'crystals' in the inner ear may cause vertigo or dizziness that can be easily investigated.

# Malfunction of the Medulla Oblongata

This part of the brain connects the brain with the spinal cord. It has numerous nerve fibres connecting the brain with the rest of the body below.

This part controls the heart rate and the strength of its contraction. The rhythm and depth of respiration is controlled from here as well. These are two vital centres as without them life can not be sustained. It also has centres that control digestive juice secretion, the movement of food through the gut, swallowing, movement of vocal cords etc.

Thus when the Medulla Oblongata malfunctions you get palpitation, fainting, breathing difficulty (breathlessness), etc.

## Sum up

The Ali Syndrome is a complicated medical condition that involves understanding the inner sanctums of the brain, so it is not surprising it has evaded scientific explanation so far and is only now becoming clear as brain research advances. Its diagnosis is equally hard to comprehend and is therefore the subject of the next chapter. The main difficulty in researching The Ali Syndrome is that it has to be studied in real time in living bodies (in vivo), which is generally considered as unethical.

# Chapter 5 - Diagnosing The Ali Syndrome

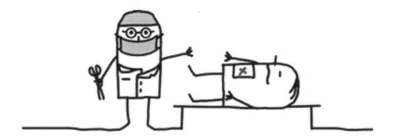

## *At least FIVE symptoms should be present to be qualified as typical of The Ali Syndrome, since there can be other individual causes…*

Thus we see that the majority of our bodily functions can be affected by the weakening of the functions of the subconscious brain. The Ali Syndrome is a series of symptoms appearing in different permutations and combinations due to lack of blood supply to the subconscious brain caused by problems of the neck. At least FIVE symptoms should be present to be qualified as typical of The Ali Syndrome, since there can be other individual causes. For example, if you just get a headache, nausea, photosensitivity and sickness, as in a migraine attack that appears before the onset of a period, then it cannot be diagnosed as The Ali Syndrome.

In a case of Chronic Fatigue Syndrome, however, with symptoms like fatigue, muzzy head, headaches, sleep disturbances (jet-lag type sleep), dizziness, short-term memory loss, lack of concentration, depression, lack of motivation, craving for sugar, palpitation, panic attacks, a poor immune system, cold hands and feet etc, then The Ali Syndrome can be diagnosed. In fact, a typical CFS is almost certainly The Ali Syndrome if trauma to the head and neck precede the onset of these symptoms. It is essential to establish that the lack of blood flow to the subconscious brain, due to the conditions of the neck mentioned earlier, has been the primary cause. For example, if you get viral infections of the brain or nerves, such as Epstein

Barr or other viruses, then the same symptoms may also prevail (as in ME or post-viral fatigue) when it is not The Ali Syndrome: The neck has to be involved in vast majority of cases.

On physical examination of the neck, one should find tender points on one or the other side of the neck. If probed carefully, some protrusions can be found along the side of the vertebrae. These hard 'lumps' are sore to touch. The protrusions are due to misaligned cervical vertebrae. Sometimes pressing on these protrusions can cause a headache on the corresponding side. This may sometimes cause tinnitus (a loud noise in the ear).

If the person is asked to move the head sideways towards the left and right shoulder for 5-10 times, he or she, will experience dizziness to some degree. In severe displacement of the vertebrae, the dizziness will be more pronounced. Sometimes, this causes some degree of nausea, blurred vision and imbalance. This is a universal test for The Ali Syndrome. The dizziness caused by movement of the neck is an indication that there is an obstruction of the blood flow to the Cerebellum, caused by misalignment in the neck. One may argue that this could be an inner ear problem. In order to exclude that, I ask the person to bend the head forward and backward for 5-10 times to its maximum point. If there is dizziness, then the inner ear is the cause. Lateral movement puts maximum pressure on the arteries and this reduces the blood flow even further.

It is best to go through the checklist for a range of symptoms that constitute The Ali Syndrome. The more positive symptoms there are, the more sure you can be that you have the syndrome.

Some other, less convincing, tests are soreness in the area of the occiput, in the back of the skull, where the tendons of the neck muscles are attached. Further questioning may be necessary: Do you feel fatigue or dizziness in a crowded place, like the metro or a crowded bar, in a smoky environment, when you are in steam room or when you inhale petrol fumes or wet paint? Do you feel sick when driving on winding country roads? Do you sleep with the windows open and keep your face out of the duvet or blanket?

Do you feel clear-headed when you are in fresh air? Does mountain air make you less tired or dizzy or sick? Have you had an accident, birth injury or whiplash? Do you use computer a lot?

All the above questions can confirm that reduced oxygen supply to the brain makes the symptoms more intense. Stagnant air makes you worse, whilst fresh air makes you feel better.

If you see asymmetry of the face (one eye more shut than the other, one side of the mouth drops), you can deduce that there was lack of blood flow to the brain due to neck problem or arterial spasm.

Another relevant question is 'Do you feel tired and sleepy immediately after a meal?' If blood flow to the brain is already restricted, the formation of a blood depot around the stomach and intestines after meals deprives the subconscious brain of more blood/oxygen. This causes extreme fatigue and dizziness.

If you get "muzzy head", extreme fatigue, nervousness etc shortly after drinking white wine or champagne, which are absorbed very quickly, the chances are that you suffer from The Ali Syndrome. To metabolise this alcohol, the oxygen in blood is quickly utilized. This depletion of oxygen causes the brain to react strangely.

A similar situation occurs just before a period when there is pelvic congestion. Women have worse PMS (Premenstrual Syndrome) when they have neck problems and when they suffer from The Ali Syndrome.

The following conditions make the symptoms of the Ali Syndrome more pronounced:

- Dehydration (reduces blood volume)
- Anaemia (reduces Haemoglobin or iron)
- Low blood pressure
- Excessive sweating (causes loss of salt)
- Candida infection in the gut, which produces toxic alcohol in the gut and so there is already an underlying fatigue
- The use of recreational drugs or excessive alcohol consumption

- Altitude
- Chronic diarrhoea
- Osteoporosis
- Deficiency of hormones, including Thyroxine, testosterone, oestrogen (as in menopause)
- Diabetes
- Chronic underlying illness such as cancer
- Alcoholism
- Chronic fever
- Respiratory disease (Asthma)
- Smoking (20 or more cigarettes a day)
- Clinical depression/Anorexia

## Self Diagnosis

One can self-diagnose The Ali Syndrome. When I used to write a weekly column in the YOU magazine with the Mail on Sunday, I used to mention The Ali Syndrome. Some doctors criticised me by email but those patients who suffered from it could easily identify the cluster of core symptoms that go together as a complex. I often had patients who would come to me and say 'I think I have got the Ali Syndrome.'

In 'Dr Ali's Ultimate Back Book', published in 2002, I wrote a chapter called 'The Neck Connection', referring to my discovery. This book sold many copies and I had patients with The Ali Syndrome saying 'it seems you have described my illness.' It is an accurate assessment of this condition.

To summarize, here is a comprehensive list of all the symptoms which constitute The Ali Syndrome (you can be diagnosed as having The Ali Syndrome only if you have FIVE of these symptoms):

- Chronic fatigue
- Breathlessness on exertion (not related to heart and lung disease)

- Headaches, both general or one-sided
- Dizziness or vertigo
- Nausea
- Sickness with vomiting
- Palpitation (an increased heart rate)
- Hyperventilation (breathlessness)
- Panic attacks
- Cravings for carbohydrates - sugar in particular
- Short-term memory loss
- Jet-lag type sleep patterns (awake at night and tired during the day)
- Lack of concentration and often absent-mindedness
- Lack of comprehension (feeling 'blank')
- Tinnitus (ringing in the ears)
- Weak immune system with frequent coughs and colds
- Allergic reactions (Eczema, asthma)
- Autoimmune Disease, including Rheumatoid Arthritis, Psoriasis, Lupus
- Extreme intolerance to white wine and Champagne
- Rosacea (redness in the cheeks)
- Mellasma (dark pigmentation on the face or skin)
- Facial paralysis on one side (Bell's Palsy)\
- Severe pain on one side of the face (Trigeminal Neuralgia)
- Blurred vision or loss of field vision (some)
- Painful joints and muscles (Polymyalgia Rheumatica - auto-immune disease)
- Food intolerances
- Retarded growth in teenagers
- Lack of periods (Amenorrhoea)
- Aggravated menopausal symptoms (hot flushes, anxiety)
- Unexplained infertility

- Nervous tic on the face
- Burning sensation in the face, neck, torso
- Burning sensation in the arms, thighs, feet (sympathetic nervous Dystonia)\
- Accentuated smell (strong smell)
- Depression (not clinical depression, which is a disease)
- Double vision
- Loss of the sense of smell or taste after an accident or trauma
- Burning mouth syndrome (on the tongue and palate)
- Loss of libido and Impotence
- Irregular periods
- Loss of periods after stress, trauma or a whiplash injury
- Irregular periods, weight gain (Polycystic Ovarian Syndrome)
- Spasm in the throat as if choking (Globus Hystericus)
- Premature Puberty (before 10 years of age)
- Cold hands and feet and also chilblains
- Blotchy skin
- Fainting - in extreme cases (syncope)
- Grinding teeth whilst asleep (Bruxism)
- Sleep Apnoea (intermittent breathing)
- Restless legs at night
- Narcolepsy (abnormally long sleep)
- White glove-like hands which are freezing cold (Reynaud's Syndrome)
- Hypersensitive skin on one side of the face or arms
- Water Retention
- Fatigue after meals and PMS or PMT
- Imbalance
- Car or motion sickness
- Mild Hypertension (Blood Pressure)
- Weight gain

- Macular degeneration (loss of vision due to age or after accidents), Cerebral palsy (spasticity in the body, retarded milestones)
- Epileptic fits after head and neck injury
- Possibly Autism, Dyslexia if related to birth injuries

In hypothalamic malfunction, there is a test that can be used to prove it. Take a blunt tipped object, such as a used biro, paper cutter, fork and scratch two parallel lines on the inner surface of the forearm. Wait for a few seconds. If the scratch lines turn red, then everything is fine. However, if it is pale and does not turn red in a minute, then the Hypothalamus, which is the controller of the tone of smaller blood vessels, is malfunctioning. The pressure on the blood vessels under the skin flattens them, hence the pale colour. Normally, the vessels will spring back and dilate to allow more blood through a natural reflex action. The lines turn red. If the capillaries fail to respond and go into spasm, then they turn pale and this is indicative of a lack of a message from the Hypothalamus.

Sometimes, there is an abnormal response after a couple of minutes. The two scratch lines remain very pale but on either side the blood vessels dilate. Thus you see four red lines and two pale lines. This is also due to an abnormal response from the circulatory control system of the Hypothalamus.

This test is termed 'positive' when the scratch lines remain pale. It means that parts of the Hypothalamus and indeed the Sympathetic Nervous System, (the Autonomous or involuntary nervous system) are not functioning very well.

This is an indirect way of proving the malfunction of the subconscious brain, which causes The Ali Syndrome. Visual proof with blotchy pink 'marble' like skin on the arms is another test. The blood vessels constrict or dilate under the skin to create this 'blotchy' look. Then you can touch the left and right half of the skull or face. If one side feels more sensitive than the other, then the presence of the symptoms of The Ali Syndrome is very likely. This difference in sensation is probably due to the lack of blood flow to the root of the 5th cranial (Trigeminal) Nerve. The roots are thick and are fed by tiny blood vessels of the Basilar-Vertebral arteries.

This is the sensory nerve for the face and part of the scalp.

If the person with the Ali Syndrome is emotional or enters a warm stuffy room, the cheeks turn pink. The Hypothalamus mistakenly 'thinks 'that the body is over-heated and so sends instructions to dilate blood vessels, which are plenty in the cheek area, to radiate heat. In fact cold hands and feet but flushed or warm cheeks, is a positive indication of the Ali Syndrome,

## Variations in symptoms of The Ali Syndrome

The million-dollar question is why some symptoms of The Ali Syndrome are more prominent or noticeable than others? Reduced blood volume decreases its pressure and depending on the genetically determined anatomy of the various blood vessels, some areas are more starved than others. Then there is this phenomenon of the 'Law of Dominance', as I call it. If you have several damaged root canals in the teeth, the worst of them will hurt first. One strong symptom will dominate the others. If you have vertigo, the chances are you will feel nauseous, anxious and panicky but your pain in your tooth will be suppressed. The body likes to deal with a few symptoms at a time. Some conditions like low thyroid, poor immunity, rheumatoid arthritis etc may gradually manifest themselves over a period of time and may not be identified in the initial stage.

People have varying threshold levels for pain, discomfort, dizziness, depression etc Strong-minded people or those who have very demanding or responsible jobs, tend to override their symptoms more easily. Some have a 'Get on with it' attitude to life. Symptoms like headaches, fever, fatigue vertigo, imbalance etc make them lose their confidence and then they seek a doctor's help. If one gets Bell's palsy (paralysis of one half of the face), then one is very alarmed. It is on the face and so people will constantly ask "what happened to you?". They feel embarrassed.

## Acute or Chronic?

Although most symptoms of the Ali Syndrome are chronic or manifest themselves over a period of time, an acute attack can also happen. Vaso-vagal Reaction is one of them. When an acute or sudden loss of blood supply to the subconscious brain causes a person to have a black-out and faint. Such patients even see the 'shrouding darkness' coming just before fainting, though they often don't remember this. Acute dehydration, a crowded place, hot sun, sudden stress from the delivery of bad news etc can trigger this reaction. You just have to lay the sufferer flat on their back, massage the neck gently and stretch it and they will revive. A drink of water or sweetened juice will replenish the energy supply to the brain.

The most intolerable symptom of The Ali Syndrome is Cluster Headaches, (very painful headaches) especially when you get them every day, all of the time for three months or so and vertigo, when you sway to one side and collapse as the world around you spins in one or the other direction. You have total loss of control. My technique has come to the rescue of many such patients.

## Exclusions of The Ali Syndrome

The symptoms I have mentioned are the most common ones associated with The Ali Syndrome. There are many symptoms which have been excluded in the above list. The subconscious brain regulates everything in the body and so many more symptoms can be found. Hypoglycaemia (drop in blood sugar), autoimmune diseases such as Vitiligo, alopecia, Schogren's disease (with dry mouth and eyes), Parkinsonism, essential tremors (in the hands and head) etc have been deliberately excluded because I have not been successful in curing them using my techniques. They must be linked to the Hypothalamic-Pituitary axis and that is only a logical conclusion.

The subconscious brain is a very complicated part of the brain. One still doesn't know all of its functions. I guess it controls our very existence and so when there is power failure in this region, anything can happen.

# <u>Chapter 6 - Exploring The Ali Syndrome</u>

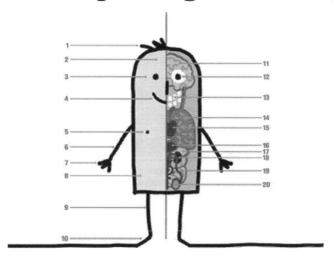

## Chronic Fatigue Syndrome (CFS), a typical Ali Syndrome

CFS is probably the most classic example of The Ali Syndrome. It can display many of the symptoms mentioned earlier. I call this 'the Power Failure of the body'. It's as if someone has turned down the life force. Besides fatigue, the main symptom, there is an entire range of symptoms such as headaches, dizziness, nausea, lack of motivation, short-term memory loss, jet-lag sleep, lack of concentration, a 'muzzy' or 'foggy' head, as if you are absorbed in a TV programme and you are not in the world around you, loss of libido, dysfunctional periods in women, body-ache from loss of muscle tone, palpitation, a poor immune system. One has to have 80% of the above symptoms to be classified as a sufferer of CFS.

When one is run down and the immune system weakens, one is likely to contract the Epstein Barr virus (the Glandular Fever virus). This virus attacks the lymphatic glands nerve and muscle tissue causing devastating fatigue. This condition is called ME (Myalgic Encephalomyelitis), otherwise known as Post-viral Fatigue. All the above symptoms prevail except that the viral infection makes them more prominent.

Since a poor immune system, caused by neck tension and exhaustion, precedes the viral infection, ME is regarded as a severe form of the Ali Syndrome. Since ME is a post-viral fatigue, the antiviral treatment is not effective in its aftermath.

## Treatment of CFS at high Altitude: My own experiments

I have been using my techniques at an altitude of up to 1500 metres to treat CFS and other conditions for the past 22 years or so. Sportsmen and army personnel often train at altitude to improve their stamina. The results obtained after the treatment of CFS patients at altitude is even more convincing. Firstly, patients adapt to a different environment, culture, food, sounds, colours, and the life of people of the Himalayan region. Then the body has to adapt to the altitude although at this altitude the body is put through some stress but there are no uncomfortable symptoms like dizziness, headaches, palpitation etc

Patients with CFS go through a programme of yoga, walking for 2-4 hours in the valley or mountains, diet and most importantly, my massage technique. The walks are graded so that one walks on different gradients or for longer, each day. The fatigue from walking and aches caused by the strain on the joints and lactic acid in the muscles is eliminated through massage. One therefore feels fresh each morning. In the morning the yoga asanas refresh the mind and invigorate the body. This programme is done over a period of ten days or so. The patients notice the change in their condition and become more confident. Some walk additionally in the evening and continue to feel very energetic. This helps to remove the burden of being tired all the time. This new found energy creates a very positive 'feel-good' factor.

In the late 80s when I started this altitude therapy, I carried out blood tests before and after treatment. The average increase in Haemoglobin levels was 0.5gms and there was an increase in Red Blood Cells. At high altitude, the body obviously needs oxygen but its supply in the air is low. The yoga and walking forces the body to produce more haemoglobin in the blood, so that more oxygen can be supplied to the tissues. The neck treatment improves the blood supply to the subconscious brain, which further improves energy levels and boots the immune system.

Pollution in cities and urban areas, I have noticed, lengthens the treatment of CFS. In fact, patients treated at altitude feel very tired for a few days after returning to polluted places. Then, after adaptation, the energy comes back. This is when they are encouraged to go to the gym, walk in fresh air or to spend weekends in hilly places. The benefits achieved at altitude helps the body to heal itself in a few weeks. This is how CFS sufferers are rehabilitated in their mind and body.

## PET Scans (prove that poor oxygen supply to brain causes CFS)

There is a special type of investigation called a PET (Positron Emission Topography) scan, where radioactive glucose is injected in the blood and then a series of photos are taken to see how they are distributed. If a part of the brain or body, doesn't receive enough blood, the concentration of this glucose, in those particular tissues, will be reduced.

In California, PET scans of the brain were done in patients with CFS. It showed hypo-perfusion (reduced supply) of blood in the brain tissue in over 65% of cases. The results published did not specify whether the subconscious part of the brain was more affected in patients. I am confident that if such a study were repeated, my hypothesis could be proved right.

PET scans are expensive and uncomfortable, as the head needs to be fixed for imaging. Sometimes the scans may take a long time to do and that is disturbing for those who are claustrophobic and have to go into a machine.

## Headaches

I will have to specify that under this heading all headaches, except for migraine, will be covered. All migraines are headaches but not all headaches are migraines.

Headache is a symptom which can be caused by various factors. The most common cause is the impaired blood flow to the brain due to neck problems. All osteopaths and chiropractors will also confirm this because, within seconds of neck manipulation, the patient will be relieved of a headache. This happens in the vast majority of cases.

## Non-Ali Syndrome Headaches

There are categories of headaches which do not respond to the therapy that improves blood flow to the brain. These causes of headaches are not related to the neck. If one has a frontal headache in the forehead, it is most likely to be due to sinus congestion. You may have a clear nose, but the sinuses are often packed with thick mucus which may occasionally drip down the throat. This is termed as 'Post Nasal Drip'. To treat it you have to avoid mucus producing foods, such as dairy, ice creams, sorbets etc My sinus oil, containing sesame, mustard and eucalyptus oils, dropped into the nostrils and sniffed, helps to de-congest 'blocked' sinuses. The headache then disappears.

If one clenches the jaw, grinds one's teeth at night, eats a lot of nuts or hard meat, one is likely to get arthritis or inflammation, of the jaw joint (TMJ – Temporomandibular Joint)) located in front of the ear. This joint becomes very sore to touch and the pain from this joint can irradiate to the temples, mimicking a one-sided headache. It is often confused with the half-sided neck type of headaches experienced by the majority of sufferers. Massage the affected joint, with some balm or oil, for a few minutes and the headaches will disappear almost instantly.

Headaches due to High Blood Pressure are usually felt in the back of the head in the occiput area. Treat the BP problem and the headache disappears. Sometimes with injured ligaments and tendons in the occipital region, say after a whiplash injury, one can experience an ache which mimics a headache. Massage the area affected or sore areas in the back of the head with balm or oil and the pain will disappear.

Headaches in the crown of the head are often due to increased fluid pressure in the brain. There could be a variety of reasons, from stress, insomnia, high BP, meningitis to tumours. Please consult a doctor. In fact, if the headaches do not disappear after the treatments mentioned in this section you must consult a doctor for scans and a diagnosis.

If you have pain in the front of the head, especially when you try to read, then you need to have your eyesight checked. The eye muscles may be strained and you might require glasses or eye exercises to sort that out.

## Ali Syndrome Headache as one of the minimum FIVE symptoms

The most common form of headache is one-sided and with a neck problem on the corresponding side. If you suffer from frequent headaches, say more than once a week, which last up to a day and without sickness or photophobia (light sensitivity), then the chances are that some vertebrae on that side of the neck are misaligned. There could be a ligament or tendon injury in the area between the occiput at the back of the skull and the neck. Press these areas with your fingers and they will be painful. My massage-manipulative technique will help to eliminate such headaches.

The neck-type of headache is frequently associated with chronic fatigue, dizziness, muzzy head, palpitation and other symptoms of The Ali Syndrome.

## Migraine

Migraine is a syndrome which involves vomiting, nausea, sensitivity to light or sound, intense half-sided headaches which last for 2-3days before settling down on their own and is periodic in nature, often occurring in women just before menstruation begins.

In my opinion, migraine is like flu. It can heal on its own within 3 days. It is as if there is some imbalance in the body and when the balance is self-restored, the symptoms disappear. The migraine headache is very strong and has a devastating effect on both the mind and the body. People generally resort to strong painkillers or anti-migraine drugs, which makes the blood less viscous so that it can flow with ease through the vessels to reach the brain tissue. Soon after taking these drugs, the pain disappears, but as the effect wears-off it returns with the same intensity. You need to repeat the intake of such drugs so that, after 3 days or so, it disappears completely on its own.

My main approach is to prepare the body in between migraine attacks, so that the blood flow to the brain is uninterrupted and thus, when they do come, the episode is mild or bearable or there is a longer gap between them. In this case, it is important to have the treatment regularly for 3-4 months, when the headaches go. I have treated numerous cases of migraine in my 30 years of practice.

# Summary

This description of the Ali Syndrome is probably best summed up by a description of actual cases I have treated using the technique.

## Constant "cluster headaches" – every day for 3 months or more

My late friend, the film producer, Ismail Merchant (*Howards' End, Room with a View*), recommended me to an Arab gentleman, from a very respected family, because of his constant cluster headaches. This is a form of headache which happens once a year, especially in the spring to early summer period - more commonly in men. The headaches will be there daily, for a month or so, continuously. For the entire period the sufferer is debilitated and nothing except strong migraine pills and oxygen helps.

Anyway, the gentleman sent his plane to collect me from Stansted Airport in London, UK and I arrived at the destination late at night. Next morning, I saw him at 10 am and saw that he had an oxygen cylinder near him. The headaches were so severe that only oxygen helped him. No painkillers worked. I felt so sorry to see him with such pain. The very first question I asked was about any accident he had had. He was quite surprised, because he had had an accident when his four-wheel drive rolled over several times in the Arabian sand dunes, some four years prior to my visit. He immediately recalled that he had started getting headaches shortly after the accident. He hadn't linked the two and no doctor had asked him that question. He had seen specialists from various places, but none knew the cause of his headaches.

I touched his neck and it was extremely sore on the right side and so was the TMJ in front of the right jaw. He clenched his jaw whenever he had the pain from his headaches. He had not used the oxygen that morning and had a certain degree of pain. This pain went shortly after my treatment. That afternoon, he followed his passion and took his boat out to sea; dived for half an hour and fed the sharks.

I did visit him a few times and he had one of his therapists repeat the treatments daily. This treatment stopped the headaches. I had advised him to have regular treatments throughout the year. He had a spa area at his beach house and the therapists were from the Far East. This helped him to have less frequent headaches with less intensity. He did not need oxygen and life was comfortable. Cluster headaches are generally difficult to cure but in this case he went into remission.

## Twice a week headache, for years

Angela, from the Midlands in UK, had headaches for 40 years, since childhood. She used to get headaches at least twice a week and lived on painkillers. She had read my column in The Mail on Sunday a UK Newspaper, where I answered the question from a headache sufferer and so she sought my advice as a last resort. I asked if she had dizziness, neck tension, fainting bouts as a teenager, along with nausea, irritability, lack of concentration, fatigue and sugar cravings. She answered 'yes' to all these symptoms. I then asked her if she had a birth injury and she immediately said that her mother had an almost 24 hours long and difficult labour. At the end forceps were used. She also had hurt her neck from some falls.

Angela came down to see me every week for four weeks and then twice a month for 3-4 months for treatment. That was the end of her headaches. She found a local sports massage therapist, whom she sees regularly. I have not seen her for almost ten years now. Menopause can cure the hormone-related monthly migraines, but frequent headaches like hers are cured only with increased blood supply to the brain.

## Headaches on every Saturday night for two days in a row

A well-known chef in the UK used to get headaches every Saturday night at 11pm. He would return home early from his restaurant every Saturday as he expected the headache. He would get tightness in the neck, followed by a severe headache. He hated taking medicines for headaches but he saw no alternative. He would continue to have headaches on Sundays as well and feel absolutely fine by the evening. He had had allergy tests, but nothing showed any concrete evidence that they caused the headaches.

I put him on a diet that excluded yeast products, dairy, coffee, nuts, sugar, citrus fruits and alcohol. I saw him on Fridays. At first the intensity of headaches lessened and then he began not to have a headache on Saturdays. Today, he is free from headaches. I see him frequently on television and once, at a conference, I heard him talk about his headaches and he gave me credit for teaching him the right diet and for applying the exact treatment.

# Dizziness and Vertigo

Dizziness is a milder version of vertigo which is a condition with a tendency to whirling. You feel as if your surroundings are moving around you. If you turn round and round in one spot and suddenly stop, the world around you seems to move and you loose balance.

Dizziness or giddiness, is becoming more common due to stress, excessive computer use, driving, flying in aircrafts with uncomfortable headrests, changing pillows due to frequent travelling etc With the slightest movement of the head one experiences these symptoms.

Vertigo is a violent attack of extreme dizziness. The eyes roll and you lose balance and can collapse on the floor, unless you hold onto something to prevent it from happening. You get very panicky, the heart races, you sweat profusely etc Sometimes, you feel as if you are going to pass out. I have experienced it once myself.

## My own experience

In 1988, I went to the Lakshwadeep islands, close to the Maldives with the Indian Presidential Party as I was treating the First Lady for a condition. A special village was built with pre-fabricated houses and I had one right on the beach. The President, with his officials, went about their engagements. I asked the Naval officers, who were there for security reasons, if they could take me snorkelling.

A high-speed rubber dingy arrived and took me to an area with pristine coral reefs. I put on the glasses and the tube and jumped into the sea. What I saw was paradise. A big fish swam past me. The corals and the sea world, with numerous varieties of fish were so beautiful. I was totally engrossed in that world. As I was warned that there were sharks in these waters, I was on the lookout. When I bent my neck to look ahead, my eyes went dark and my limbs were numb. Then, suddenly, I felt the sea churning around me. The Naval Officer saw me going limp and jumped into the water. We were all in our skin suits. He pulled me onto the boat. The vertigo was very scary. I thought I was going to die. As the boat rocked, it felt worse but with some presence of mind, I began to squeeze my neck with my hands. Somehow, I managed to tell them to lie me flat with my head right down and to massage my neck and shoulder. Once horizontal, I felt slightly better, but very nervous. The Naval Officer panicked and started the boat to take me back to the shore. I think he tried to radio the medical post, but I told them what it was and they calmed down. My neck was very sore and the jumpy movements of the small boat over the waves made the situation worse.

They took the boat right up to my unit; I staggered across the beach and peeled my clothes off. I lay on my back and asked the Naval Officer to give my neck a pull. They were so kind and did what I asked of them. If I hadn't been a doctor, I am sure I would have landed-up in the Medical Inspection Room. After only a few minutes, I felt calmer. I continued to breathe very slowly, holding my breath for up to 15 seconds and my heart rate came down. I felt extremely sleepy. I lay on the floor and asked the officers to leave after thanking them for their help.

I had been busy on that Presidential Tour. We went to Cochin in the Southern India from Delhi and spent the night there, flew in helicopters to a naval ship, had lunch with the entire crew, slept in cabins with a strong smell of diesel; saw naval exercises on high seas with aircrafts, mock fights, helicopter rescues, sonar detection of submarines etc It was great fun watching the exercises with The President of India and his family, but it was no doubt very exhausting, especially as I had to do treatments as well. I hardly slept at night because of uncomfortable beds and different environments.

All that tightened my neck and the sudden movement of the head must have misaligned a vertebra in my neck, causing an acute reduction in blood flow to my brain. Fortunately, I knew what it was and organised my own treatment. I was well by the evening and attended a folk dance performance on the makeshift helipad. The news of my illness was revealed to the Presidential Party and they were all very concerned. I felt embarrassed, as I was the doctor. That evening in the officer's mess where the senior officers dined, we had a good laugh. Later that evening, when I went to see the First Lady, she asked me what had happened. News does spread fast.

## Long hours on computers leading to neck spasm

The secretary of an important Arab dignitary and businessman in the Middle East, worked long hours on computers. He suffered from insomnia and had had an unhealthy lifestyle for several years at a stretch. It started off as fatigue, headaches, slight dizziness, blurred vision and short-tem memory loss. As time went by, he began to get palpitations. One day, while driving on the main highway, he had an extreme attack of vertigo. He swerved the car sideways onto the grass verge, flung open the door and lay flat on the ground. He began to shake violently, as if he was having an epileptic fit. Some people gathered round and took him to hospital.

After a lot of investigations, including brain scans, nothing substantial showed-up. He was put on a tablet for vertigo and it was diagnosed as an inner ear problem. This is the most common diagnosis for extreme dizziness and vertigo.

I was in the country on a routine visit. I examined him and my diagnosis was the lack of blood flow to the cerebellum, due to extreme tightness of the neck muscles. His boss half-believed my diagnosis and gave me the benefit of the doubt. As requested, he joined me with a group of patients on one of my health trips to a remote castle in Rajasthan in India.

He responded positively to treatment and he felt very relaxed and energetic. One day we had to take a 3 hour bus journey on a bumpy road. He fell asleep on the bus and had his neck in an awkward position. When we reached the castle, he tried to get up but had another attack of vertigo. His eyes moved rapidly, as if following the whirling of the world around him and he was almost unconscious. He then had a mild seizure. I had just got off the bus when this happened. I went back and had him lie on his back in the passageway and immediately began to work on his neck. I gave it a bit of traction with my hands. As soon as he felt a bit better he tried to get up but had another attack of vertigo. He panicked, as do the majority of people in this situation. It is very scary, as you feel you are going to die.

There wasn't a stretcher, as it is a remote castle. I used a blanket and, with the help of a few people, carried him to his room- the round gun room – where, 300 years ago, stood the main cannon that defended the fort from invaders. We had the maestro, Ustad Sultan Khan, a very well known musician in the group, who played an ancient instrument called the Sarangi, a stringed instrument which is played with a bow, it is very similar to a small Cello. Without any hesitation, he sat in the centre of this large, round room with a dome and began to play a tune. The sound of the Sarangi is very similar to the human singing voice. As my patient lay flat on his back, without a pillow, I gave him some water to drink, with the help of a tablespoon. He could not lift his head, lest it triggered another attack.

I gently treated his neck and felt the misalignment of the neck vertebrae. Sultan Khan's music was divine when it echoed in the domed room. I have never treated anyone in such superb ambiance. I was totally enchanted by the music of one of the geniuses of Indian classical music. My patient drifted-off into a deep state of relaxation. About half an hour later, he got-up to use the toilet. It was miraculous. The notes of the Sarangi had enhanced the therapeutic effect of my treatment a thousand times.

Next morning he was in the courtyard talking to a few people in the group who were enquiring how he felt. He was calm and relaxed, joking with everyone. It was impossible to imaging the situation he was in the previous evening. His treatment continued and he is now totally cured. I met him seven years later; he had taken a couple of years off to study, but he had returned to his job. He never had another vertigo attack again.

## Extreme vertigo and imbalance

A dear friend of mine, Silas Chou, whom I have known for over twenty-five years, owned a very successful garment business. Some of the labels are, like Tommy Hilfiger and now Michael Kors, world famous. One morning, after his routine jogging, he felt extreme vertigo and collapsed on the floor. His wife called me immediately and I contacted Dr Nachi, a friend at The Harley Street Clinic in London, UK and he kindly rushed to Chester Square, where my friend lived. He was admitted to The Charing Cross Hospital. He was diagnosed with an inner ear problem. I knew it was his neck that was responsible for the vertigo attack. He flew regularly to New York and Hong Kong on his private jet. We used to say that he lived on his plane and he only landed, from time to time, to stretch his legs. He was known to jog on runways while his plane refuelled.

I went to the hospital and his face looked pale. He was on medication and his darling wife Cecile looked every concerned. I explained how neck stiffness can restrict blood flow to the brain, sometimes acutely after some violent movement (in his case after jogging). They knew about my theory and no convincing was necessary. I massaged his neck, which was extremely sore to touch. When he felt better, another mild episode started when he tried to get-up to go to the toilet. I made him lie flat on his back and continued treatment for over 2 hours until he fell asleep.

CT scans of the brain and inner ear were taken and some other tests, which involved water and a tilted bed, were carried out. There was some grit or crystals, found in the ear. In this case, there was a problem with the ear as well as the neck condition. He was discharged from hospital and I gave him more treatments at home. He began to fly again. He also had some more tests in America and the inner ear disease called Meniere's disease was diagnosed. I told him to have regular neck massages and exercises. He travels much less now and has not had any more attacks. As friends we meet each other from time to time, even though he lives in New York.

My question is that if crystals in the inner ear caused it, why was it so acute and only happened for one short period of a few days? I agree that Stugeron or Stemetil are drugs that suppress car sickness, dizziness and vertigo, but they don't actually cure them. Silas changed his lifestyle; had regular neck and shoulder massages, as instructed, and does regular exercises. He is now cured.

# Imbalance in Elderly people

Elderly people suffer frequently from imbalance. They feel that the floor is swaying as if in an earthquake. They begin to walk awkwardly, fixing their eyes on the surface on which they walk. This changes their posture and they often develop a 'hunch back'. They often shuffle their feet and that is sometimes mistaken as Parkinsonism.

## Degenerative keen joint

A former Prime Minster of a major democratic country walked very slowly and shuffled his feet. Tests showed he had a degenerative keen joint and so everyone thought he couldn't walk because of his knee. A top surgeon from the US was called in and his knee was replaced but walking did not improve, even after many months of physiotherapy. I was invited to see him. At first glance, I could tell he had imbalance. Moving his head from left to right a few times cause dizziness. I made him stand, close his eyes and told him to walk. He lost his balance and nearly fell down. This is a typical test for imbalance.

 I discussed his imbalance with his doctor, a leading orthopaedic surgeon in that country but he didn't believe me. I asked the patient about accidents. He quietly told that as a teenager he wrestled a lot and was dropped on his neck and shoulders numerous times in the sand.

I suggested treatment under my care that gave him relief but he was still slow and so didn't walk much as he was old. What followed later was heartbreaking. The advanced complications of the neck connection followed. After a few years he had a stroke and was bed ridded. I heard that he has lost his memory and has signs of dementia. It is very sad because he was a bright man, a writer and a poet. He was well-respected politician of this populous democracy. I wish the treatment had continued under my supervision.

## Motion Sickness on boats or in a car on winding roads

This is an extremely unpleasant sensation and includes dizziness, headaches, sweating, flushing of the face, nausea, vomiting and mood alterations. At first, sufferers may feel the excitement of giddiness with palpitation, but then they have extreme disgust and can even feel suicidal. It happens when the body (head) moves in a car or on a ship that rocks or tilts from side to side in the sea. In rough seas almost everyone gets these symptoms.

The eyes play a part in balance control. They fathom the height of the head from the ground and the distances of objects around you in order to adjust your posture, so that you don't fall. So when you rotate your body in one place or go on a merry-go-round, your balance is upset for a few minutes after stopping. The eyes see objects go round in quick succession. When you stand on a wall to jump down, you are scared because your body's height is added to the height of the wall and therefore, you feel much higher than you actually are. It is a greater height than you could actually jump from and you then sit on the wall to reduce the total height and jump.

For sea-sickness, which is a part of motion sickness, sailors will tell you to look at the horizon and fix your eyes there and not on the sea, which is tilting sideways all the time. Fixing the eyes also stabilizes the neck. This reduces the risk of vertebral arteries compression due to lateral movement of the neck.. Some patients, who go with me to the Himalayas for my health programme, get car sickness due to the winding roads. The car constantly turns to the left and then to the right. The road to Shimla has notorious turns and bends, as it was built for slow moving cars and horse carriages. The British went up to the hills from Delhi for almost nine months a year to beat the heat of the plains. It was the summer capital of India. Today's fast cars make the journey very unpleasant and people prefer the small train journey.

I have noticed that on my Himalayan trips to higher altitudes, the neck massage and manipulation helps people to cope much better with both motion and altitude sickness. For example, in the beginning motion sickness in some people would be horrendous. I advise them to fix their eyes on a distant point on the road and not to look out of the window. This is difficult, as the scenery is spectacular. Some close their eyes and sleep. This helps. After a few days, with regular treatments, which all patients have, the motion sickness improves. If you have smaller meals the vomiting then reduces, but the nausea remains the same. I give the vulnerable people anti-sickness pills and even antihistamines with strong sedative properties. This knocks them out for a while and when they wake-up, they don't panic and the journey becomes much easier. In the early days, when we used a bus for our Himalayan journey, my staff would give the guests neck massages every hour or so. This would tremendously help those who were susceptible to fatigue, muzzy head and car sickness.

## Phobia of getting into a car because of dizziness

A lady in her seventies began to get a phobia of getting into a car. Every time the car accelerated or braked, she felt nauseous. She lived in central London, where the traffic is erratic; it made her movements within town almost impossible. I had treated her for headaches and dizziness already. I was aware of her chronic constipation, which caused poor calcium absorption, as this element, along with magnesium, is predominantly absorbed in the colon. She later had osteoporosis due to calcium deficiency, as a result of which the neck shrank a little. This aggravated her circulatory problems. I treated her constipation, gave high quality coral calcium in water, massaged her neck regularly and gave her some exercises. After a few sessions, her symptoms disappeared. She had spent a lot of time and money investigating the problem, even though the solution was simple. She felt comfortable in a car after that.

# Ringing in the ears (Tinnitus)

Tinnitus is the hearing of noises where there is no sound in the surrounding environment. This noise could be buzzing (bee, mosquito or bumble-bee sounds), ringing (a constant ringing of a bell), a steam engine or pulsating sound, corresponding to the heart rate or pulse, a high-pitched noise or whistling and all the variations of these sounds. A loud bang or noise at rock concerts and discotheques can also kick-start tinnitus. In this case the noise 'damages' the sensitive hearing nerve endings in the cochlear-part of the inner ear.

I must confess, unless someone with tinnitus comes to me within 6 months of its onset, I cannot do much to eliminate it. When I treat tinnitus using my techniques, especially in the early days, the sound disappears soon after the session. They can bring it on simply by thinking about it. I always tell them to keep the 'sound' out of their mind, once it disappears after the treatment session. This part is extremely difficult because some people get very agitated with the constant ringing or buzzing. It is said that Van Gogh had tinnitus and the sound irritated him so much that he cut off his ear. Meditation, deep breathing and sound sleep helps to push the thought of the sound into the background. The treatment helps to diminish the sound, but one has to use will power to keep that away. It's better not to remind oneself of the sound altogether.

I sometimes recommend Ginko Biloba and B-Complex, in addition to the neck treatment, in order to facilitate recovery in the early stages of the disease. The neck treatment should be done professionally once a week for 8 weeks or so, but the patient should also self-massage the neck, the jaw on the affected side and the area below the base of the ear. This area is extremely sore in people with the Ali Syndrome. Massage gently for 3-4 minutes and then deeply for another 4 minutes. It's best when someone else does the treatment, especially when everything is so sensitive to touch.

Sometimes blocked ears, due to a closed Eustachian Tube which connects the middle ear to the throat, can exacerbate the symptoms. In that case, put 2 drops of my sinus oil or sesame oil, into the nostrils and sniff. After a couple of minutes, try to 'pop' the ears, as you would in an aeroplane. For some this 'pop' will not happen immediately and so you have to try, morning and evening, for several days until the tube opens-up.

Almost immediately after 'popping', the hearing improves. So, if one suffers from slight hearing loss (which is not caused by nerve damage, an explosion or punctured ear drum) as well as tinnitus, which is often the case, the hearing- loss masks tinnitus and is pushed to the background. You need to keep the sinus decongested and the Eustachian tubes clear by avoiding cheese, ice cream, chilled drinks, cream, yoghurt and excess sugar. Also, make sure the bowels move regularly, by drinking more water (at least 6-8 glasses per day); eat figs, papaya, prunes, spinach, beetroot etc Chronic constipation causes the sinuses to become congested due to a toxic mucous discharge.

Conventional medical treatment is limited to using a special hearing aid that produces a more acceptable sound to mask the unpleasant and irritating noises. Acupuncture has been successful in a limited number of cases.

In my opinion, the auditory nerve or hearing nerve, which comprises of the vestibular (for balance) and the cochlear part (for hearing), is a thick nerve. Branches of the vertebro-basilar artery feed it. Tinnitus especially that which is not caused by sound damage, responds better with improved blood supply to the nerve root through these arteries. This is limited to the ringing or whistling type of tinnitus. After disembarking from a long-haul flight, one often has fatigue, a muzzy head, along with mild tinnitus. Perhaps this is from constant engine noise over a period of time. A good therapeutic massage after the flight and ample rest and rehydration, eliminates tinnitus quickly. Sometimes those who live in noisy urban areas experience tinnitus when they go to the countryside for the weekend or holiday, which is much quieter. There is a residual noise in the ears for a couple of days. Once rested, the noise disappears. The vertebral artery after emerging from the protected canal of the neck vertebrae makes a loop before entering the brain. This loop is located just below the hearing apparatus of the ear. Plaque deposits in the vertebral artery may cause turbulence and produce a rhythmic sound. This sound, which corresponds to the heartbeat or pulse, has a periodic 'whooshing' tone. This type of tinnitus does not respond to neck treatments, as the cause is mechanical and not related to the nerve. This is an actual not virtual sound.

Some people hear a fairly constant 'popping' sound. This is usually due to the partially blocked Eustachian tube letting in air into the middle ear. As I mentioned earlier, this tube originates in the upper part of the throat and connects with the middle ear. Its main purpose is to blow the walls of the middle ear to form a chamber, in which three tiny bones are located. One lies behind the ear drum and the other lies in front of the window of the inner ear, which picks-up the vibration of sound and transfers it to the nerve endings. The middle bone connects these two other bones. These bones simply transfer the vibrations of the ear drum to the auditory nerve. Mechanical vibration is thus converted into electrical impulses, interpreted as sound.

When the Eustachian tube is blocked, due to a throat or middle ear infection, the bones in the middle ear cannot vibrate efficiently. This leads to hearing loss, as sound waves are not sent to the nerve ending of the inner ear.

My advice is that Tinnitus can become chronic. It rarely goes without treatment and it is an annoying condition, especially when you focus on it all the time. Stay calm and ask someone to massage your neck before you seek professional help from a trained therapist. Check the treatment method described later in this book.

## Buried under the rubble for three hours with severe neck injury

A friend of mine was in a hotel New Delhi, which collapsed after a large terrorist bomb explosion. He was buried under the rubble for three hours. He was with his girlfriend, who sadly died lying next to him. He had a lot of damage to the neck vertebrae, a couple of which had to be surgically fused. For years he had suffered from severe headaches, dizziness, nausea, tinnitus, deafness, anxiety, insomnia, chronic fatigue etc; in fact, he had full-blown Ali Syndrome. Most of the symptoms went away with my treatment, but tinnitus and deafness remains. He is used to it now and leads a normal life.

## Tinnitus after whiplash injury

The owner of a garment chain in London had Tinnitus a few months after a car accident. It disturbed him very much as the noise was high-pitched and continuous. Someone recommended him to see me. He said he would do anything to get rid of it. I gave him frequent treatments. He did the yoga exercises; followed a diet with no excess salt, sugar and coffee to calm down his nerves. It worked quite quickly. His tinnitus disappeared, only to return after a long-haul flight. He came back to me immediately and it was resolved again. After a few episodes, it stopped. He understood the trigger and began to manage it well.

# Nausea and Sickness

If you are anaemic, the oxygen supply to the brain is restricted due to lack of Haemoglobin. This causes fatigue, slight nausea and breathlessness on exertion. All these symptoms get worse when you smell wet paint, petrol fumes or walk into a crowded place or smoky environment. The oxygen in the air is reduced in these conditions and so you feel very nauseous or sick; sickness is a result of extreme nausea. You yawn a lot to get more air.

Similarly, when the neck restricts blood supply to the subconscious brain, nausea or sickness are common symptoms, especially when you move. If the oxygen level is low in the environment, the nausea materialises into vomiting. During my high altitude journeys across the Indian Himalayas with groups of patients, nausea, sickness and vomiting were common symptoms. Every year since 1994, I have had to spend more time in Manali (7000 feet) to acclimatize. Then in 2003, I took my therapists along and we needed just 3 days of acclimatization at 9000 feet. After the treatments, all the 12 participants, including one who had had part of her lung removed due to cancer, crossed the Bhaba Pass which is at an elevation of 16,500 feet. For the first time, all of us had the breathlessness, but no sickness. The only variable was the special neck treatment. After that, I included this treatment on every trip and no one has had any problems with the altitude since.

Sickness is the body's own way of elimination of fluids from the gut. As a result of that, the body gets dehydrated and the blood becomes 'thicker'. There is more haemoglobin per ml of blood, so more oxygen can be absorbed. Temporarily, this fixes the problem of oxygen supply to the brain; thicker blood means more oxygen concentration.

## Projectile vomiting in a child with neck injury

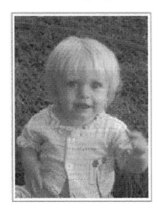

I was visiting my friends Gaynor and Johann Rupert in South Africa for Christmas and New Year. On Christmas Day, I saw a little girl Chloe of nine months who was brought to me. Chloe was the daughter of their Farm Manager, Mark in the Karoo. She looked pale and her hands and feet were cold. The parents drove down for several hours to see me and were very anxious. She had a tiny feeding tube in her stomach. For six months she had projectile vomiting after every feed. She could not retain anything. She had a few operations and was fed upside down to let the food go up the stomach. By the way, in the head down position, the sickness stopped as the brain got more blood. The mother discovered a method of feeding her intuitively. They were told she had multiple food intolerances and nothing concrete could be done. She was hospitalised over 10 times but no solution could be found. She also suffered from frequent bladder infection, was nauseous along with gagging and retching. She was tired and slept a lot as a result of chronic fatigue. The doctor finally thought she was 'neurotic'. They prescribed antidepressants.

I asked her parents about her birth. She was a caesarean baby. I then asked if there had been a fall or accident. At first they couldn't recall any trauma. My brain ticked to find the right clue. I touched her neck and she was visibly uncomfortable. I started massaging the neck and her parents were getting concerned as their baby began to cry. Suddenly her mother recalled the trauma. When she was three months old and lying in bed, her elder sister jumped on her and she had cried a lot after that. The nausea and vomiting started shortly after that. There was a direct, definite link between the trauma and symptoms.

I then explained what had happened. The trauma had affected her neck and so she had problems with blood flow to the brain. This had caused the fatigue, nausea, retching and a poor immune system (hence the frequent bladder infections). It sounded like Greek to them, but they gave me a chance. After fifteen minutes of treatment of the neck, jaw, throat, scalp, shoulders and upper back, her face turned pink and her cheeks were red. I said that was because the blood was flowing into the head. This convinced the parents of my diagnosis, as she had always been so pale.

Next morning, they came to see me. Her mother was very excited as the baby had drunk 50 mls of milk for the first time without vomiting. They always thought she was allergic to milk. She had been on formula milk since she was only three days old. That was a big relief, as I needed the parents' faith and cooperation. I wanted them to massage her neck 2-3 times a day.

I taught them the technique and massaged the mother's neck to demonstrate the appropriate pressure and technique.

I saw the baby for a week. Everyday there was something new to report. They kept in touch with me via email and sent me photos of her progress. She has grown to be a delightful child; active, chatty and even a little mischievous. The feeding tube was removed and she now eats everything. I expect her to grow up to be a tall girl. As I will explain later, by stimulating the Pituitary gland with a proper blood supply, the secretion of the growth hormone increases which boosts a growth spurt.

## Sickness after eating, leading to sever weight loss

A lady from a highly respected family in the UK had suffered from sickness for over nine months. She had lost almost three stones in weight. Every possible test had been done, but nothing substantially wrong could be found. Her family was extremely worried. The doctors had diagnosed it as a psychological problem. She had been given all sorts of tablets. After every meal she would be sick and sometimes even drinking water would produce the same result.

Initially, the doctors looked for stomach ulcers and then viral gastritis. They desperately tried to find a proper cause or diagnoses. Sadly, a lot of drugs had been prescribed which not only suppressed the appetite, but also made her zombie-like, which was picked-up as depression. The weight loss did not help, as she became very tired and malnourished. She would eat small meals, 6-10 a day, and sometimes she could retain only a small amount of that food. That sustained her basic energy.

I was asked to go and see her. She lived alone in the country, but her daughter had come down to assist with all the further arrangements.

I examined her tongue and she looked dehydrated. Some vertebrae in the neck were misaligned. I asked her to move her head sideways for five times and that caused dizziness. All the telltale signs of the neck connection were there.

Then I asked her about an accident she might have had. She said she had none. I gave her some hints, and asked if she slipped on the pavement and fell. She recalled immediately that, three years previously she had fallen very badly in her house. The carpet near the stairs did not have any grippers and so she slipped on the wooden floor. She had hit the back of her head and had concussion. Afterwards, she had some headaches and dizziness.

I explained what had happened. She couldn't understand the link, but wanted to give the treatment a try. After the first couple of treatments, she responded well and her appetite returned. I told her to eat soft nutritious foods. She ate pureed vegetables, mashed potatoes, mushy rice, minced meat, grilled or steamed fish, fresh juices, cottage cheese, porridge etc she avoided citric juices, so that there would be no gastric irritation. She began to recover slowly and the nausea and sickness stopped.

## The Emotional Element

I was always fascinated by Psychiatry as a subject. Even when I was about twelve, I used to go to the American Library in Calcutta in India, during my holidays from my boarding school, to read books on this subject. In the final year of my MD course in Moscow, I used to spend my free time and do night duties in Hospital No 8, a Psychiatric Institute. I was very interested in Anorexia Nervosa, which was beginning to spread amongst young women in the former Soviet Union. I did a paper for the Student's Scientific Society, almost like a mini-thesis, comparing the condition with a mild form of Schizophrenia. Critics will now disagree, but in those days it was well accepted.

As I mentioned earlier, when blood flow is reduced to the brain, people can get various psychological and emotional problems. A slight reduction of blood flow tends to produce symptoms like fatigue, drowsiness, lethargy, depression, sighing, "sinking feeling in the head.", lack of motivation, lack of concentration, feeling "detached" (as if watching a TV film where you are not participating), zombie feeling, fear etc. A more moderate decrease in blood flow will produce anxiety, panic attacks, irritability, lack of reasoning, excessive talking, phobias (in chronic condition), being excessively suspicious, obsessiveness, hyperactivity, "high-pitched" voice, severe insomnia. Severe restriction of blood can cause severe panic attacks, tremor, fainting, fits and other more pronounced reactions like marine attacks.

The above symptoms are subjective and cannot be measured unless on a scale of 1 to 10 to assess the severity. They are generally treated under "psychological and emotional" problems. Antidepressants, tranquillisers, sedatives are used to "mask" the symptoms so that people can carry on with their lives without affecting the people around them with their unreasonable behaviour.

## Depression as part of The Ali Syndrome and Clinical Depression

I must clarify that depression is a very common symptom prevalent in society. There are two types of this condition. The first is a symptom of the Ali Syndrome where lack of blood flow is the primary cause. You reinstate the blood flow and the symptoms are reversed. The other more serious condition is Clinical Depression which is an organic disease. Here, the disease is deep-rooted. The lack of neurochemicals, like serotonin, is a noticeable marker of this disease. Unless these chemicals are replaced, the Depression as a disease cannot be cured. Similarly, if lack of insulin gives Type I diabetes, it is essential to inject the hormone to keep the blood sugar in check. Hormone replacement therapy is essential for Thyroid malfunction, as for Ovarian, Testicular or Adrenal malfunctions.

In Clinical Depression, the symptoms are more pronounced. People cry, have morbid thoughts, even of suicide, feeling of listlessness and total lack of motivation or decision-making capacity. Such patients can't work and are stubborn in their thoughts. There is no way my neck treatment will cure that. It can help to give some relief.

## Emotional and other problems after physical abuse in childhood

A young lady came to see me with full-blown Ali Syndrome symptoms. She had chronic fatigue, dull headache, jet lag-type sleep disturbances, (tired during the day, awake at night), lack of concentration, dizziness, hormonal imbalance (severe acne, in her 30s, facial hair, dark pigmentation on the skin, low thyroid function), craving for sugar, palpitations, hyperventilation, blurred vision, occasional tinnitus, intolerance to wet paint or petrol fumes etc Additionally, she had severe panic attacks, restless leg syndrome at night in her sleep (tossing and turning), vivid dreams (almost awake), screaming, sleep-walking, Bruxism (grinding of teeth) in her sleep; multiple phobias (flying, insects, dirty toilets, claustrophobia. She also had a fear of following pregnant, even when she was in her safe period, frequent mood swings and severe premenstrual syndrome, lasting for two weeks before the periods. She couldn't work as she hated everything in the office. She felt suffocated and hated her colleagues. Additionally, she had Crohn's disease (an autoimmune disorder), which gave her abdominal cramps, diarrhoea; bloating etc I asked her if she had any injuries. She couldn't recall any. I gave her hints like car or motorbike accidents, falls, excessive dental work, knock on the head, swimming pool accidents etc She couldn't recall any such traumas to the head and neck. When I asked her about being hit on the head by someone, she broke down and it took a large part of the allocated consultation time to calm her down. In childhood she was beaten very badly by her mother, who even once tried to strangle her. She was slapped and her head was banged against the wall on several occasions. Then her boyfriend was violent as well. I could clearly see the picture.

I wrote down everything for her, as she had short-term memory loss. I showed her the model of the neck and a section of the brain and explained her the functions of the limbic system (responsible for emotions, sleep, motivation, moods), the hypothalamic-pituitary area (responsible for the hormonal imbalance, palpitations, Crohn's Disease etc), and other parts of the subconscious brain responsible for many of her symptoms. She immediately said she had extreme neck tension and discomfort. She had dizziness when I asked her to move her head to the left and right. She believed in my explanation.

A couple of days later, I gave her a neck treatment and gently manipulated it. She had instant rush of blood to the head. She flushed and said that the room looked brighter. She began to cry as she was overwhelmed with emotions.

After a few treatments, she felt a lot better. She opened up and began to tell me more about her personal life. She started yoga, changed her diet and had weekly neck treatments. Today she is a transformed woman. Her skin, her energy, her moods, her periods, her concentration, her digestion and her outlook towards life have improved. She began to apply for jobs and even thinks of starting a business.

## Drug and Alcohol Addiction

I often wondered if my treatment would influence drug and alcohol addiction. I took several patients of cocaine, marijuana, alcohol and social drug addiction. A young woman with a successful career was addicted to cocaine. She was instructed to give up cocaine. She received a daily 2-hour neck and body massage. She drank soup and fresh vegetable juice, water, herbal tea and my Detox Tea. As expected, she felt very drowsy and slept for up to 16 hours a day in the first few days. Cocaine makes you "awake" so its withdrawal causes drowsiness. After a week, she felt a lot better.

I sent her to the Himalayas to the place where I usually treat chronic patients. She had massage, did yoga and walked in the mountains every day. Some of the walks were tough, and she often complained of fatigue. My assistant would encourage and motivate her to walk further. Every time she would climb atop a hill, she would be encouraged to say. "I can do it; it's not difficult for me anymore". This gave her the positive affirmation. The feel-good factor created by the neck treatment played a very positive role. She is now off drugs for 5 years, with a good chance, forever.

In alcohol addiction too, similar treatments can help a lot. The diet/juices help the liver to Detox. Neck massage creates the energy and feel-good factor and walking in the mountains, helps to build willpower. With a determined effort, supported by a boost in energy, addicts are able to quit their habits.

## Eating Disorders

When I moved to London from Hong Kong in 1991, I became aware that eating disorders were quite common the UK. Bulimia and binging were quite widespread. Those who suffer from this condition, feel quite 'full' after eating. As they eat fast and excessively, they feel tired and slightly nauseous. It is because if this feeling, some make themselves sick. The nausea, in some women, is definitely a trigger point. The ritual of forced vomiting then becomes conditioned and they do it after every major meal.

I came up with the idea of my neck treatment to stop the nausea after meals. After a heavy meal, the blood rushes to the abdomen to aid digestion (the secretion of juices, the churning of food, the movement of digested matter further down the GI tract), which is a taxing mechanical process. When that happens, the brain is deprived of blood. If one has severe neck problems, the blood flow to the brain is reduced even further, so the nausea becomes more prominent.

## Bulimia: forceful sickness after sickness

The daughter of a successful Asian businessman from Bombay, India went to a boarding school in England. She missed home and so had depression. When she was sixteen years old, she became bulimic. She managed to hide it from her family during her holidays in India.

She approached me. I began to give her neck massages, taught her yoga, gave her some herbal antacids and gave her some tips on relaxation. I also told her to lie down flat, without a pillow, soon after a meal so that the blood could flow to her brain with more ease. This integrated approach began to help. Her nausea after meals reduced and then disappeared. She usually fell asleep after meals. When she woke-up after a nap, she didn't feel the need to be sick. That was my first case of bulimia and my system worked. Today she is married and has children.

## Psychological aversion to food: Anorexia Nervosa

A couple of years ago a beautiful lady, in her mid-forties came to see me with fatigue and insomnia. She had had several horse-riding and skiing accidents and also suffered with headaches, nausea and palpitations. I suggested she went on my Himalayan Programme for treatment for Chronic Fatigue Syndrome. She made child-care arrangements for her children and booked onto the trip.

In the Himalayas, I noticed she was very fidgety. She would eat quite a lot and then walk about in the dining room feeling quite restless. After a week, I asked her why she looked so disturbed. She then told me the real story.

As a teenager, she was anorexic but with time she got better. After a few years she had a lot of stress and she became bulimic. She suffered for fifteen years and even though her nausea and urge to be sick reduced in the Himalayas. The abdominal muscles contracted involuntarily after meals, as if she was retching. This was a disturbing feeling and it was for this reason she was so restless. She started to attend the meditation classes in the evening. The neck massage, yoga and meditation gave her the strength to overcome a long battle with bulimia. Not all patients with bulimia can be treated like this. Some will need serious psychological treatment.

# Cravings for sugar or food

The appetite centre is located in the Hypothalamus, which tells us when we are hungry. It also tells us when we are full so that we can stop eating. The feeling of satiety is also obtained from the stomach muscles being stretched to their maximum capacity.

If the glucose level in the blood drops, the appetite centre gets panicky, as the brain needs fuel all the time. One gets irritated and some even get headaches when hungry. Furthermore, if neck problems restrict blood flow to the Hypothalamus, the craving for food is more prominent. Finally, when the stomach is empty the accumulation of acid in it irritates the nerve endings on its walls, creating hunger pangs. The more acid you have the more you want to eat. So, on an empty stomach, in people with neck problems, food cravings are very strong. If you don't see food on the plate you get very upset. Thus the expression 'a hungry man is an angry man'.

Craving for sugar or sweets, is more prominent with stress, excessive computer use, insomnia, lengthy drives, in premenstrual period etc because of neck tension. After a meal, when blood rushes to the abdomen, the glucose supply to the Appetite Centre in the Hypothalamus is reduced. Additionally, if you have a neck condition, the cravings become unbearable. Many people crave for something sweet a few minutes after a meal. That is why desserts are served at the end of a meal. Sugar suppresses the craving immediately.

When one gets cravings for sugar or one is very hungry, a small amount of sugar can suppress the craving and you don't need an entire chocolate bar to achieve this! What happens is that the sweet-tasting buds on the tongue pick-up the signal and sends it to the Hypothalamus, which then sends the message to the liver to release stored glucose. The sugar (sucrose) one eats cannot be digested immediately, as it takes a while to be split into glucose by digestive enzymes. Only glucose can be utilized as 'fuel' in the body.

You can use this phenomenon to temporarily stop your food cravings. Take a polo mint or a couple of raisins and you will feel the cravings subside as soon as you put them into your mouth.

Food, especially sugar cravings, is one of the many causes of weight gain. Those who have problems with binging have the worst form of psychologically-induced cravings. They will secretly buy or store chocolates, fruit bars, sweets etc some cannot resist sweet shops. The traders, too, prey on such people. They display a variety of chocolates, sweets, bars etc of all different brands. Even though the main ingredient is sugar, cocoa, butter etc the chemical flavourings alter the taste to cater to the individual's needs. It is just like the different brands of cigarettes on display,

In my weight loss plan, which I am using in the Castel Monastero and MITA Resort Srl, Italy Spa in, Tuscany, the main aim is to control or suppress, the appetite. This is done firstly by reducing stomach acid production. Those who eat very fast, use a lot of chillies, drink a lot of orange or lemon or pineapple or grapefruit juices, white wine, alcohol etc have excess stomach acid. This increases the appetite. Secondly, by allowing the taste buds to function better, the feeling of satiety comes sooner so people are encouraged to eat slowly. Thirdly, the neck massage helps to keep the glucose supply to the appetite centre in the brain under control. Finally, my herbal teas suppress the appetite.

## Binging and weight gain

A friend's secretary was desperate to lose weight. She lost her boyfriend, could not fit into her clothes and hated herself in the mirror. She had tried the Atkin's Diet; lost quite a bit, but put it back on when she stopped the programme. She couldn't keep up with her exercises as she became fatigued easily. Her boss, my friend, asked her to see me. She felt embarrassed, as she had to disclose her problems to me. She couldn't handle it.

Finally, one day she made an appointment to come and see me. She started talking about her ankle sprain, backache, chronic fatigue and occasional headaches. I went straight to the point: did she binge? She finally admitted that she craved sugar and sweets all the time. I tried to discover if she had any trauma to her head or neck. She couldn't recall anything, but admitted that she worked long hours in front of a computer and used two pillows to sleep. The neck stiffness was the main cause of her symptoms.

With an excuse to treat her neck and back, I gave her some treatment. After a couple of sessions, I asked her if her sugar cravings had reduced. Her eyes twinkled with surprise; the cravings had disappeared.

I explained why she had them and put her on my weight loss plan. Without her cravings, her weight dropped and she was strong enough to go to the gym 2-3 times a week. She was ecstatic. Everyone, including me told her how wonderful she looked. That boosted her morale enormously. The more weight she lost, the better she felt. It was difficult to believe that this lady had transformed herself so well. The sugar and food cravings had imprisoned her.

## The roles of oxygen and glucose in brain function

If lack of oxygen in the environment causes fatigue, headaches, dizziness, fainting etc then lack of glucose in the blood or hypoglycaemia causes panic, emotional problems, shivering, cold sweats, disorientation etc The body has reserve of glucose and so a sudden release of stored glucose eases the situation. It is when that reserve is exhausted in extreme cases that the body experiences serious symptoms like fainting, coma etc

Oxygen is mainly supplied to the brain by the blood, whereas glucose is also provided by the cerebro-spinal fluid (CSF) which bathes the brain

During clinical fasting, patients undergo treatment for 15-20 days or more, with just water and a little honey. No food is given to them and the body is forced to release fuel from stored fat in the body. Thus, lack of glucose in the brain tissue is not fatal but lack of oxygen has serious consequences. In an acute stroke, the body becomes paralysed on one side often with loss of speech or swallowing and consciousness. The blood clot totally starves the corresponding area of oxygen, causing nerve cells to fail. Oxygen is absolutely essential for the functioning of the brain cells.

# Paralysis of one half of the face (Bell's Palsy)

This is a condition where one half of the face becomes paralyzed. The eye is wide open; the angle of the mouth drops and the tongue is forked on one side.

This happens as a result of the loss of function in the facial nerve or 7th Cranial nerve, which originates in the midbrain. Most physicians or neurologists, think that the condition is a viral infection of the facial nerve or due to inflammation of the nerve by or cold draft on that side of the face.

This is the main nerve for the facial or mimicry muscles, controlling one's expression. A part of the nerve picks up information from the taste buds in the anterior part of the tongue (which tastes both sweet and salty flavours). Besides this, the branches of the facial nerve control the secretion of tears, mucus discharge in the nose and salivary secretion.

My hypothesis is that the Basilar Artery, which is formed by the joining of the two vertebral arteries from left and right sides, has branches that feed the roots of the facial nerves. These blood vessels are tiny and are called vasa nervorum (vessels of the nerve).

When the pressure of the blood in the Basilar Artery drops, due to constriction in the vertebral arteries, the vasa nervorum receives very little blood. This impairs the function of the facial nerve and the result is Bell's palsy.

It is very frightening, as within a few minutes, half of the face becomes non-functional. It is not a stroke and one has ever found a virus in the nerve, but I have all the necessary proof to confirm that it is due to impaired blood flow to the facial nerve. By restoring the blood flow with my neck massage and of the facial muscles, along with exercises, the functions have been restored in hundreds of cases.

## Early treatment of facial paralysis (Bell's Palsy)

Tom Chapman, the son of my close family friends Frank and Wendy Chapman woke-up one morning with his face paralyzed on one side. The worst symptom was his inability to close his eyelid on the affected side and his speech was impaired because of the inhibited tongue. He went to his doctor who prescribed him steroids, which is standard medical treatment. He panicked because he was in the fashion business and had to deal with elite customers. Tom owned 'Matches' a well known luxury chain for clothes in London.

Tom came to see me late that night at home. I reassured him that he would be alright and explained exactly what I thought had happened. He had been extremely stressed because of the business, had an unhealthy lifestyle, travelled a lot and had slept badly. His neck was very stiff as expected. I saw him regularly for a few weeks and the symptoms disappeared.

## Facial Paralysis in a teenager

The teenaged daughter of a dear friend, Stephen Marks whom I have known for over 22 years, suddenly had Bell's palsy. She panicked and began to cry a lot. Stephen who owns French Connection fashion chain is one of my great admirers. He brought her immediately to see me and I assured her that she would be cured. I gave her a couple of sessions of neck treatment and taught her nanny to continue with the treatment while they were on vacation in St. Barts in the West Indies. After about 10 days, she came back to see me, smiling and very happy. As I had known her since she was a baby, I was naturally very pleased to see her in high spirits.

## Hectic life, fatigue and stress leading to facial paralysis

The President of a major world institution was travelling a lot and was very exhausted. One afternoon he told his secretary to cancel his post-luncheon appointments as he was very tired and didn't have the energy to meet anyone. He lay on the sofa in his large office and slept with a cushion under his neck. Within minutes he drifted-off into a deep sleep.

When he woke-up, one half of his face felt strange. He got-up and felt dizzy and imbalanced. He called his secretary who was shocked to see him. He was pale and the facial expression on ᵗᵈe had gone. She immediately called the emergency services.

The helicopter ambulance landed on the top of his office block and he was taken to the best hospital in Washington DC. A CT scan and all other tests were done. There was nothing wrong with his brain and heart as it was a classic case of Bell's palsy.

Steroids were prescribed and physiotherapy was recommended. With rest, his fatigue improved, but the face remained lop-sided. The word spread and the Chinese Government sent their best acupuncturist to treat him, as he was very important for the development of that country in the nineties and also because he was a very well-respected leader of that institution.

The acupuncturist treated him for five weeks, following him around on his plane. His face improved slightly and he was able to partially close his eyes. He didn't feel right about his condition, as he was a public figure and was frequently photographed. Most people who met him asked what had happened and he found that very embarrassing.

A senior member of the British Royal Family met him in his Washington office for some work. Seeing him, he immediately recommended me. He very kindly sang my praises and described my work with stroke research at The Hammersmith Hospital in London, using my technique. I received a call to say that I would be called from the office of this important gentleman in Washington who had Bell's palsy.

I was in Geneva, in the beautiful Beau Rivage Hotel, when I received the call from Washington. The gentleman asked me if I treated a late case of Bell's palsy, as five months had already passed and he had not fully recovered. His eye did not shut properly and it watered very often. I told him about my theory and technique which he found quite interesting. He wanted to fly me over to Washington DC. I explained that I was treating someone in Geneva and would be available the following week

He suggested that I flew to New York the following weekend and go on to join him in Aspen, Colorado, where he would be available for three days. He had no major appointments there, other than sit on a panel, and would therefore be available for five days in all for treatment. This was the only clear slot in his hectic schedule.

I flew to New York, had supper with him in his beautiful apartment on Fifth Avenue and went to La Guardia airport. On his plane, after take-off, I began to treat him on his bed, as I did not want to waste any time. Being a small Lear jet, it was slightly cramped, but I had adequate space to treat his neck, face and then his entire body for over two hours.

His neck muscles were extremely tight, as I expected. He too was very surprised, as no one had ever noticed that. I could feel that a couple of vertebrae in his neck were misaligned. I warned him that he would hurt slightly because his neck was stiff. Time was short and I had to condense the treatments. When I treated his back and his legs, he felt relaxed and fell asleep. I was then able to recline in my seat and relax.

We stayed in the house of Evelyn and Leonard Lauder of Esteelauder, the cosmetic family. They were such a wonderful couple. The following morning, my patient came down and said he felt slightly better in the face and certainly more energetic. The improved blood flow to the brain had done the trick.

We went to the conference venue. Ted Forstman, of Gulfstream organised this conference every year and invited all the aircraft owners for a three-day event. Major speakers were invited to share their views on the economy, politics, environmental issues etc I met many world statesmen and important people there like Colin Powell, George Schultz etc. The conference was fabulously organised and the speakers were excellent. I learnt so much from the discussions. Then there was a surprise! President Nelson Mandela was linked via satellite and he spoke to us from Cape Town. That made my day, as I adore Mandela. Years later, I had dinner with him once organized by my friends Ruperts of South Africa.

After lunch, I would go for walks with Leonard and Evelyn in the wild mountains. With renewed energy and a refreshed mind, I treated my patient twice a day. My patient became more confident. He saw the truth behind the 'Neck Connection'.

I managed to treat him again on the plane. I showed him all the exercises; drew the diagrams for his physiotherapists, so that he could continue his treatment in America. He did come over to London a couple of times and I gave him treatment in his hotel. His condition steadily improved. In his case, the physiotherapy and acupuncture made the initial improvement but that soon reached a plateau and he made no further progress. My technique and treatment pushed the progress up from the plateau. I wish I had seen him right from the beginning, and then he would not have had to go through that agony for so many months.

From time to time, I have seen his photograph in magazines and I study his facial expressions. It did look almost alright, except for a slight droop in the angle of his mouth.

# Complication of Ageing

T.S. Eliot, the famous poet, wrote: *My life is light, waiting for the death wind, like a feather on the back of my hand.* This concept of playing out time has become out dated as technology has put power into the hands of the Elderly. As a result the population of the elderly is growing in the West. There is no "medicine" for the elderly, preventative or therapeutic. All we have is Geriatric Medicine, available to people who are overcome with illnesses of the aged.

Having dealt with very many elderly people, I feel many of their problems are largely preventable. In a nutshell, they need to eat differently, as their digestive enzymes are no longer available in abundance, and their stomach and intestinal muscles lose the ability to churn or contract as before. Softer foods and a very light dinner eaten at sunset or shortly afterwards are highly recommended.

My neck treatment helps to keep all the vital centres functioning optimally. They are able to sustain the energy level, maintain balance and coordination of gait, digest better, and prevent dizziness, severe insomnia, neck stiffness, tinnitus, blurred vision, tremor in the hands and above all retain good memory and recall.

## Macular degeneration in an elderly

A lady in her 80s had Macular Degeneration, which reduced her central vision. She also had cold hands and feet, fatigue, dizziness and imbalance. The neck treatment improved her vision and she could see faint figures on the TV. She can now walk without dizziness and her energy is a lot better. She had Reynaud's syndrome (cold hands) but that got cured over a period of time. This is another proof that autoimmune disease can also be treated with my technique.

## Management of complications of ageing

William Kessler, a man in his 80s, has been seeing me at the clinic at regular intervals for many years. His dizziness, imbalance, short-term memory, tinnitus and fatigue are kept under control with the neck treatments. We have become great friends over the years. He has been on my Himalayan trips several times. He often tells me that my discovery of the Vertebral Arteries' role in well-being and self-healing deserves a big research and recognition for its contribution to medicine. He says that it is the safest, cheapest and the most beneficial single treatment in the world. It has a cure-all effect on the body, as healing is a deeper function of Nature. Once aroused in the body, everything else gets cured automatically. In my mind stimulating the hypothalamus, which monitors and control everything that goes on in the body is the vital factor in healing.

## Slurred speech and imbalance

Bill Bruce, a friend of mine from Scotland, whom I had not seen for a while, came to see me at the clinic a couple of years ago. I immediately noticed his slurred speech. He was surprised, as his doctor didn't pay any attention to it even though he complained about it. He said he had come to see me for his imbalance and dizziness. He had many symptoms of the Ali Syndrome and a very rigid neck.

I began to see him twice a week. He would fly down from Aberdeen and stay overnight at his club so that he could have two sessions per week. Gradually, his gait and balance improved. He even went to the Castel Monastero and MITA Resort Srl, Italy Spa in Tuscany, and followed a strict programme of diet, neck massage, walking and yoga. He looks much younger, the energy level is good, sleeps well, the memory has improved, the digestion and bowel evacuation has improved and he no longer has any joint stiffness. It has changed his life. From feeling old and "Rusty" as he called it, he is very energetic and continues to work very hard.

There are other additional benefits from having regular neck treatments in old age. As they feel very energetic, and so they can walk and carry out their routine work. They suffer from less colds and coughs as the immune system improves. I have noticed changes on the skin as well. With treatment, the ageing process slows down.

Women, who suffer from osteoporosis, usually lose calcium from the neck, vertebrae, spine and the hips or pelvic bones. They lose height as discs in the neck degenerate. They feel extremely tired and complain of constant neck tension. That is followed by headaches and dizziness or vertigo, nausea, imbalance etc.

## Severe imbalance with ageing

The widow of a famous Russian Cellist who was well know in the West, was wheelchair-bound as she had no power in her legs and severe imbalance. She herself was a very famous opera singer and ran a music academy in central Moscow. I was introduced to her by a famous Russian violinist, Maxim Vengerov, who lives in Monaco. I was back in Moscow after 25 years and was very emotional, and a lot had changed since I left in 1982 after my post graduation.

On the first day I went to the Moscow Conservatory, where this amazing lady received the Tchaikovsky award, given posthumously to her late husband for his contribution to music. She walked with a couple of men supporting her on the stage. The imbalance was so severe that she had to be put on a wheelchair afterwards.

I worked on her neck and after three days of treatment, she got her strength back. She was able to walk unaided, and no longer used the wheelchair. After a few days, I went back to see her and completed the course of treatment. She was back to work at her music academy, recruiting young students for the next academic year.

## Complications after neck injury in an elderly

A friend's mother lived in Henley, near London. She could not walk as she had extreme fatigue, dizziness, imbalance and arthritis. She had a fall and broke her neck. Although the bones healed, she continued to have many of the symptoms of the Ali Syndrome. A specialist had warned her that she must not let anyone touch her neck. I told my friend to bring her to see me so that I can personally examine her. I asked a colleague Carolyn who knows my technique to visit her twice a week. After just a month's treatment the elderly lady came to see me at the clinic. She was walking without support and felt quite energetic.

In old age there is a often plaque on the inner lining of the arteries. It is then not the misaligned vertebrae but the narrowing of the arteries, which reduces the blood flow to the brain. In such cases tinnitus, imbalance and TIA (mini-stroke like symptoms) are often common symptoms. A strict fat-free diet, neck massage, exercises and sleeping on a very flat pillow help the situation. Replacement of this artery is a very risky surgery often with fatal consequences.

# Care for the Elderly Project

It is my dream to operate A Fractional Ownership Complex for the Elderly, where people between the age of 60 and 90 years could buy units for 1 to 3 months a year. These units would be self-sufficient with easily accessible facilities like common dining room, swimming pool, and areas for therapies, recreational section, multi-faith prayer hall etc Each resident would receive 2 to 3 sessions of neck and body massage per week, attend aerobatic and elderly yoga exercises and eat as per individual requirement in the dining hall. Thus each person owning the unit would have 1 to 3 months of health care with diet, massage, exercises and walks in the fresh air. They could resolve their aches and pains, improve their digestive system, relax and sleep well. Moreover, activities like film clubs, lectures, dancing classes, excursions, painting etc, can also stimulate their brains.

# Part 2

# Case Histories

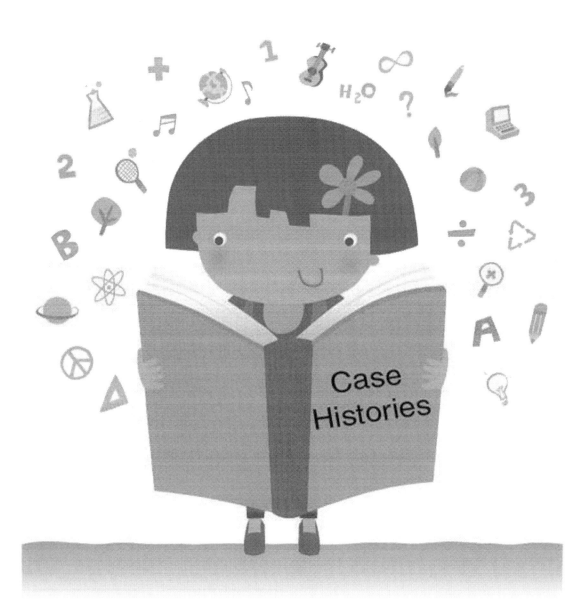

# Chapter 7 – Mini Stroke or T I A – (Transient Ischaemic Attack)

A TIA in the vertebral artery causes extreme fatigue, fainting, loss of vision, tremor or jerks and some psychological symptoms. The body may not suffer from any paralysis or weakness. It often sorts itself out.

It has all the symptoms of a stroke, like weakness or paralysis in one half- side of the body with facial paralysis on the opposite side (if the arm and leg are paralyzed on the left, the face will be paralyzed on the right), loss of speech (if right side of a right handed person's body is paralyzed), extreme fatigue etc The only difference is that it does not last long as within a few hours or days the recovery takes place, sometimes without any treatment.

For the patient or the family, it is very scary especially if the attacks occur every so often. As scans show no noticeable change in the brain it is often not considered to be serious by doctors. It is considered to be a spasm of the arteries and there is no clot formation.

A TIA in the vertebral artery causes extreme fatigue, fainting, loss of vision, tremor or jerks and some psychological symptoms. The body may not suffer from any paralysis or weakness. It often sorts itself out.

## TIA attack on a BA flight

Once I was on my way to Muscat via Abu Dhabi. I was sleeping when there was an announcement on the PA system, paging for any doctor who might be on board. I responded and a stewardess took me to the Business class section. An Asian gentleman was slumped in his seat with the face distinctly dropped on one side and was unconscious.

I laid him down on the aisle and stretched his neck. I found a few dis-aligned vertebrae in the neck and began to gently adjust them. Within a couple of minutes, he revived. He tried to get up as he was very embarrassed at what had happened. I told him to lie on his back and put a blanket under his head.

I asked his wife if he had any neck problem. She confirmed that he had often complained of dizziness and neck pain. I massaged his neck, opened his collar buttons and gave him some water to drink. After a few minutes he fell asleep. His wife said that he was very exhausted and complained of headaches a few days prior to the attack.

I went back to my seat and told the wife to let me know when he woke up. Shortly afterwards the captain called me to the cockpit and asked me what was wrong with the passenger. I explained that his neck was stiff and it cut off blood supply to the brain, causing him to collapse. Additionally, the facial nerve reacted and so there was loss of facial expression on one side. I adjusted the vertebrae of the neck and reinstated the blood flow, which revived him. He asked me if he needed to order an ambulance or medical team prior to our arrival. I said I would let him know, when we start our descent. I had suggested that landing in Tehran, as he was intending to do, would not have been a good idea.

The captain ordered tea for me gave me the duty free booklet. He asked me to choose as many items I would like to take as a token of thanks. I chose a small teddy for the daughter of a relative.

## Multiple attacks of paralysis (TIA)

A wealthy Omani businessman was in London. One evening, he had palpitation and slumped on the floor. An ambulance was called and he was rushed to a leading private hospital where scans were done and nothing could be seen. It was diagnosed as a mini-stroke or TIA. As he recovered quickly and was sent home the next day. The following evening the same thing happened and he was unconscious again so he was taken to the same hospital. This time the scan showed a massive stroke and was unconscious for a few days. It took him almost 3 years to recover and walk with a lot of difficulty. My brother Nizam was involved in the rehabilitation therapy using my technique.

TIA is often taken very lightly, especially when patients recover quickly as the blood flow is reinstated. Very often, in the aftermath, there are other attacks, some of which may be serious.

## A patient who collapsed frequently during lectures

One of the most severe cases of this attack I saw was that of a professor in Oxford University, UK. He used to collapse frequently during lectures especially if he was tired. He would lose control of his muscles of the leg and spine and slump on the podium. He had seen many specialists and no one could pin point the cause of these attacks. He came to see me in London one day.

The professor did suffer from a very tight neck and sometimes felt nervous before the lecture. He didn't have any control over the attack as he was taken by surprise every time it happened. I explained the situation and demonstrated how the neck massage was done. I suggested that he saw someone regularly for a deep tissue massage of the neck in Oxford, as the journey to London could be too strenuous for him. I showed him a set of yoga exercises too.

This professor had all the telltale signs of Ali Syndrome – fainting or collapsing, slight dizziness, long hours in front of the computer, fatigue, insomnia etc He had all the tests and scans to rule out a brain tumour, plaque in arteries, viral infection, atrophy of brain tissue etc It was Transient Ischaemic Attack or temporary attack of reduced blood supply to the brain caused by neck stiffness, aggravated by stress and perhaps an auditorium with poor ventilation. He was told it was a psychological problem that he strongly denied.

# Chapter 8 – Fainting

Massage the neck and give it a gentle traction. Give them some water to drink when they turn around and are conscious. Most people will recover and walk home but if they don't you must call for medical help.

When people faint suddenly one has to take into account some common factors. The cause could be due to anaemia or very low blood pressure, hypoglycaemia or low blood sugar, extreme fatigue, dehydration, high blood sugar (for a known diabetic), epileptic fits (when the person has a seizure), stroke etc The vast majority of them do so because of a neck condition. So if you see someone collapse in a crowded place, make the person lie on his or her back. Clear the area so that there is fresh air. Massage the neck and give it a gentle traction. Give them some water to drink when they turn around and are conscious. Most people will recover and walk home but if they don't you must call for medical help.

**Woman who had collapsed in the crowd, but not due to any neck problems**

A few years ago I was training some National Health Service (NHS) doctors in the Principles of Integrated Medical Diagnosis and Treatment in the Himalayas. One day, a medical camp was set up in a remote primary healthcare center for the doctors to examine the patients independently. When we arrived some 300 patients showed up and we were 8 doctors in all. The rumours had spread in the hills that some doctors from England were holding a free medical camp so they walked miles from their villages for consultations

We started consultations immediately. I saw a patient every 3 minutes, as sending them back home without even a brief chat would have been disheartening for them. Many were jumping the queue, as they were so anxious to see a doctor. Some had even arrived early in the morning to join the queue.

Suddenly, two of our doctors rushed to me saying there was an emergency, explaining a woman had collapsed in the crowd. I waded through the throng to reach her. She was put on the veranda, as there was no bed available. I looked at her and found her teeth clenched but she was breathing - only just. From experience I instantly knew what was wrong. I turned to the doctors, who had by then gathered there to help. 'What do you think has happened?' I asked.

They said we should take her to the nearest hospital, as the primary healthcare center was not equipped to treat her. They felt the pulse and she was breathing slowly. I was calm and wanted them to diagnose the condition but they were panicking as they thought she would die right in front of them.

I told them to come nearer and watch me treat her and I told everyone to be silent. I asked for a spoon and with it I forcefully opened her clenched teeth. They saw it was really tight. I pressed the two points in the center of the forehead, on the top of the bridge of the nose. Usually, these trigger points or pressure points, are very sensitive. When I pressed hard she blinked so I told them to observe that she responded to pain.

I moved close to her and whispered in her ears that she would be cured and there was no need to worry. I could see that the doctors were losing their patience even though they had seen mini miracles during their training programme where I showed them what could be achieved with accurate diagnosis and proper treatments. I stroked her head and massaged her jaw and the neck.

After 5 minutes of talking and using caring words, she responded and opened her eyes. The doctors began to clap and were overjoyed. They were awed by the whole incident and wondered how I could talk her out of coma. I gave the patient some water to drink and she sat up.

I called the doctors to one side and asked the medical officer of the health center to join me.

I explained what had happened, namely that it was a typical case of hysteria. We all know what being 'hysterical' means but that was a hysterical attack. It was the strongest form of "fainting" the doctors had ever seen.

In ancient times, Greek Medicine, led by Hippocrates and later by Galen, this condition was called 'hysteria' or twisting of the uterus (hystericus-uterus; hysterectomy-removal of uterus). Women who have unfulfilled sexual desire or who do not get an orgasm after severe arousal can experience disappointment and frustration. They may bottle up their feelings to avoid conflict with their husband or partner but if this happens repeatedly they develop this psychological condition. It is a great 'drama' as it tends to happen in the presence of a crowd or in family gatherings. Hysterical attacks never happen when these women are on their own. In honeymoon periods in conservative countries like India, Middle East, China etc, when young girls first experience they often don't know what an orgasm is. They are nervous and confused by the speeding heart rate, excessive sweating, tensed muscles, panic breathing etc Very often they get tremors and shakes. They can hear everything around them but cannot move and respond only to pain and smooth talking. Giving them oxygen or putting a drip in does not help as it is purely a psychological condition.

In the modern world women are sexually liberated and have gradual personal experience. Sex education helps them to know everything about it. In underdeveloped societies, such facilities are not available as sex is a taboo subject. Young girls learn from married friends, elder sisters or grandmothers. Some don't have that opportunity and so they are more likely to get hysteria. It is extremely rare phenomenon in the west.

## Sudden loss of consciousness in a crowded place

I was in the Himalayas with a group of patients, amongst who was a close friend. One evening we sat in the hall watching some traditional Indian dance performance. He was having a drink and suddenly he felt from the chair and began to shake violently almost as if he was having seizure. I lay him flat, he vomited and was semi-conscious. My nephew Ashique who knows my technique very well was there. I asked him to do the neck treatment immediately, while

I observed his pulse. An Indian minister friend who was also there asked his security office to get an ambulance and a doctor. While we waited for "emergency" help, I asked Ashique to continue with the treatment. I felt his pulse and was convinced that he would recover. I have mastered pulse diagnosis over the years. Within minutes he opened his eyes and smiled and said he was not ready to go yet. The treatment was continued and he was able to get up. We checked his blood sugar level and blood pressure just as a precaution.

I have treated people who fainted in crowded places, after emotional shock, in heat (heat stroke), acupuncture treatment, infusion therapy, blood donation, heavy periods or menstrual cramps, while fasting etc using my neck treatment.

Although the cause of fainting was not the neck but improving the blood flow to the brain helped these patients to recover quickly.

# Chapter 9 – Stroke

This is an extreme condition of cessation of blood flow in one of the arteries of the brain caused by a clot that travel from the heart to the brain. In a majority of cases the clot travels along the wider Carotid artery and plug the narrower blood vessel of the conscious brain. Depending on where the clot is and how much area of the brain it cuts out, the damage can be substantial.

The conscious or cortical brain is responsible for sensation, voluntary movement, vision, speech analysis, logic, decision-making etc. Much of it gets affected, depending on how large a clot it is. Fortunately, the other half of the brain is spared in a single stroke and so higher functions like long-term memory, recognition, analysis of the situation, communication with eyes or partial expression (if speech is gone) etc are intact or partially intact.

A blood cloth that travels through vertebral arterial network can cause death as the vital centres of the brain are cut off. A smaller clot can sneak through to cause lesser damage like loss of vision (optic nerve damage on one side) in one eye, lack of balance, vertigo etc most strokes in the vertebral arterial network are fatal. This once again proves my point. Without the vertebral arteries our existence is not possible.

Improving blood supply to the subconscious part of the brain restores such functions as breathing, heart rate, digestion, appetite, general well being, improved energy, emotions, sleep, swallowing etc This goes a long way in the general rehabilitation. It gives you the strength to go through the physical therapies and 'will to fight' is a major stimulus. Having treated hundreds of stroke victims and helped them to lead a near normal life has given me some authority to speak about Stroke Rehabilitation using The Ali Technique.

## Stroke caused by irregular heart beat

Angie Gooderham, a friend in her fifties went with me to India over the Christmas-New Year period. My mother joined me on that trip. We travelled by train from Delhi to Ajmer in Rajasthan, India, where we visited our family's Sufi shrine, offered prayers and then drove to my friend's Bijaipur castle in a remote part of eastern Rajasthan. That used to be my winter retreat until it became a very popular heritage hotel. I used to walk through the jungles looking for herbs, watching hundreds of species of birds, visiting tribal settlements to see their lives from close quarters and going on game drives with search light at night. I learnt so much about nature from being there. I learnt about the lives of ancient tribes, especially the nomadic Rewari tribe who with tens of thousands of livestock move from place to place.

After arrival we went to the terrace to look at the moon, which had a strange large halo around it. I saw Angie in tears and asked her if she was alright. She didn't reply so I thought she was overwhelmed by the peace and beauty of that 300-years-old castle. I went down to the courtyard of the castle to have tea with my friend Rao Narender Singh, the owner of the castle.

After a few minutes, one of my therapists ran down to tell me that a lady was very poorly. I rushed upstairs to her suite and upon one look I could tell that she had had a stroke that affected the right side of her body. I made the decision to treat her there as nearest hospital was in Chittorgarh, about 40 kms and Udaipur, the nearest big city was 135 kms away. Transporting her in that condition would have had its own difficulty and we could have lost her.

I began to work on the neck while my assistant worked on the Marma points that I also use to stimulate brain centers. Within a few minutes I could see the change in colour of her face and looked better.

After two hours of therapy, there was a jerk in her right leg and she could move her leg. She indicated that she wanted to go to the toilet and to my great joy and surprise, she got up to go to the toilet. It was about 10 pm. I couldn't arrange a drip as it was too late and we were in a remote village. Using a spoon we made her drink some water and she could swallow which was a great relief.

My sister- in- law Uzma who is a doctor was also there. She offered to stay by her bedside and keep her under observation. I went down to see my mother who is a very gentle and caring person and so she was terribly worried. I told her that everything was under control and Angie was feeling better.

Next morning, on the Christmas Day Angie came down four flights steps with a little help to a room on the ground floor. She had lost her speech but could just about use her right hand. It wasn't even 16 hours after the stroke and there she was sitting up in bed and smiling. She handed over a piece of paper in which she wrote a Christmas greeting for me. Some words like flavour (flower?) morning (merry?), Coming (Christmas?) didn't make any sense. That was quite amazing, as thoughts didn't translate into words.

Uzma, having worked in emergency wards, handled the case very well. She established a drip, gave her some blood thinners, plenty of fluids and organized my physical therapy every 6 hours. My mother made pigeon soup, which is a traditional remedy for stroke patients in India. She must have learnt that from her doctor father. She also massaged her feet using some form of reflexology treatment.

Angie began to improve every day. On New Year's Eve, Rao, the owner of the castle, had organized a dance performance by the Kalbelia tribe and she stood up with great enthusiasm to dance with him. I was in tears as it was one of the success stories of my life.

When she returned to London, her friend received her at the airport and took her straight to St. Mary's Hospital. A CT scan was immediately done. She had a trial fibrillation (irregular and rapid heart beat), which churned up the clot in the heart, which went straight up to the left side of the brain. I remembered that she was dehydrated as she did not drink water for the whole day because of Indian public toilets in those days, including the one in first class train coaches, weren't clean at all. The dehydration caused the irregular heart beat and the clot.

The doctor at St. Mary's could not believe that she was walking and speaking so soon after such a stroke. She called me to ask what treatment I had used and so  I invited her to come to the clinic. She never came.

## An acute stroke-recovery observed by doctors

About 8 years ago, I was training a batch of National Health Service doctors in Bijaipur Castle. One morning we went to the Chittorgarh General Hospital for a tour. We were taken to the Intensive Care Unit. There in one corner lay an old man who had had a stroke that morning and was admitted at 4am. A scan was performed earlier and the doctor in charge said he had no chance of survival. I asked him and the son of the patient if I could treat him using only my hands. They both agreed.

The patient was semi-conscious and was breathing independently. I treated his neck and shoulders using my technique and after a few minutes he opened his eyes and had tears in his eyes. The son was ecstatic, as he could not believe what he saw.

Then I began to work on the Marma points (special trigger points in the body) in the right foot and leg on his gluteal and back muscles and after testing the power of his affected leg made him sit up on the bed. When I removed my hands, he could still sit without any support. My students were very impressed with the treatment and even the doctor in the ICU, who was attending to another serious patient in the ward, came running to see this patient who was by then wide alert, sitting independently on the side of the bed.

## A late-stroke recovery observed by doctors

Later that day, we went to the Jetla Mata Temple some 8 km away from Chittorgarh in Rajasthan. This temple, it is believed, has a goddess that heals stroke, polio and paralyzed victims. I took the doctors to this temple to show hundreds of patients lying there on their own or with their family members by their side. It is amazing that some people actually get better and return home. Some don't and spend months hoping they will. The temple committee provides free food and water. Every 2 hours there is a ritual of beating drums, ringing bells and mass singing. The doctors found this whole experience fascinating.

I walked around with them and they observed the degree of disability some had. I spoke to several of them and narrated their personal story to my students. Amongst the many patients, I found an old man who had a stroke but was able to sit on his own. He was unmarried and lived on his own.

I began to treat him while the doctors watched. After a while with some help from my students, I asked him to stand. To the surprise of many, he stood up and when we let go our support he was able to do so independently. We helped him to walk a few steps and there was commotion amongst the onlookers, as they all wanted their relatives to be treated as well. It was getting late and so we had to go back to the castle.

The following day, the doctors were very keen to go back and see what happened to that man. We drove to the temple and there he was sitting down and massaging his neck and the leg with the good hand. It was prayer time and as the music and songs started some people got up to dance and chant. To our great surprise, our patient got up with great enthusiasm and began to dance as well.

A local TV crew (ETV) had heard about the "miracle" at the Chittorgarh General Hospital the previous day. When we arrived at the temple, they were already there and so began to film us. It was "Aarti" or prayer time so there were songs, music, chanting and dance. Our man stood up with a little help and begun to dance in front of the camera. It gave me immense pleasure to watch him do that.

Not all patients can make such quick recovery especially with late stroke rehabilitation. The old man needed a little power in his legs and a psychological boost. The man in the hospital was a fresh case and so response was very quick.

# My stroke rehabilitation research projects

I used my stroke rehabilitation technique in three research projects.

## Geriatric ward of the Hammersmith Hospital in London, UK

The first was at the Geriatric Ward of the Hammersmith Hospital in London in 1996 under supervision of the then consultant, Dr Mario Impalomeni, when 12 severely disabled patients with average age of 80.3 years were treated over a period of 5 months. The results amazed the team. Four walked with some aid and one walked independently.

## Stroke Rehabilitation Research at The Peninsula Medical School in Exeter in UK

The second rehabilitation research project was carried out by my brother Nizam, under the supervision of The Peninsula Medical School in Exeter in UK. That study was published in The Journal of Physical Rehabilitation in 2006.

## Stroke Rehabilitation Trial at The Mayo Hospital, in Lucknow, India

The third was done at The Mayo Hospital, in Lucknow, India under supervision of the consultant Dr Sandip Aggarwal of the King George's Medical College. Out of the selected 10 patients, 4 walked independently and 4 walked with a frame or stick. The Sahara Group headed by our family friend, Subroto Roy, sponsored the trial and organized a press conference afterwards. The journalists were baffled by what they saw and most newspapers carried the story the following day.

## Sum up

I wish I had funding to carry out further research in this area. The research team in Exeter was very keen at one time to do a large nationwide study, but funding for rehabilitation is the least of the concerns of the Medical Research Council. Unfortunately 40% of stroke victims are permanently disabled and 20% die. Only 40% regain some form of ability or are cured. Stroke is the single disease that consumes the maximum amount from the healthcare budget. These patients have to be cared for and there are millions of them. My stroke rehabilitation technique would have saved so much of money and helped many patients to live near normal life.

# Chapter 10 – Coma

This patient went on to walk, talk and be quite independent after that. The lack of blood flow to the brain after the accident was the main problem. The treatment simply reversed the process and the brain was rejuvenated again.

I worked in Delhi between 1982 and 1988 and established a good practice. Initially people were sceptical about my training and medical education in Moscow. They didn't understand Integrated Medicine and Acupuncture, Iridology, and Therapeutic Yoga etc were outside their knowledge.

## TV Documentary on Alternative Cure

With help from Mrs. Sita Murari, the wife of Mr. Bob Murari, the then secretary of The President of India, Central Television in Delhi filmed a 2- part documentary called, 'Search for an Alternative Cure'. They filmed me explaining what Integrated Medicine was and showed my work with disabled patients.

All below cases histories were demonstrated in the 2nd part of the TV documentary that was broadcast on two consecutive days after the main English news bulletin at 9 pm. It was prime time and India's only channel then broadcasting to millions of homes. Within a couple of days thousands of patients, some in wheelchairs came to see me at The Center of Integrated Medicine in Delhi. I was stunned by the response the TV programme had. My landlord and the Housing Association, run by ex-army personnel got very alarmed as lift was blocked and the residents complained. I was in serious trouble. Finally, the Housing Association forcefully closed my clinic after an emergency meeting of the committee.

I desperately looked for alternative premises but no one was ready to let one to me for fear that they would have to fight legal battles to evict me if I didn't voluntarily leave. After 2 months of search and with no place to practice from, I left India to take up a job at The Vital Life Centre in Hong Kong where I was already well- known, thanks to Aileen Bridgewater, a prominent radio talk show hostess who in just one interview on her Talk show made me famous overnight.

## Coma after a road traffic accident

The son of an Indian Diplomat was crossing the road when a speeding bus knocked him down. He was in AIIMS, India's leading research and teaching hospital for six months and was treated under eminent Neuro-physician Dr Banerjee. When his condition was status quo, he was discharged home to spend rest of his life in that comatose state. His sister, a journalist heard of me and requested me to treat him. My assistant treated him using my technique at home. One day, the sister came to my clinic with a cassette recorder. She asked me to listen to the recording and it was my patient uttering his first words, quite incoherently. She was ecstatic. This patient went on to walk, talk and be quite independent after that. The lack of blood flow to the brain after the accident was the main problem. The treatment simply reversed the process and the brain was rejuvenated again.

## Coma after brain surgery

The daughter of a senior staff member in St. Columbus School (I studied in a similar Christian Brother's School) went into a coma after a brain surgery to remove a tumor. She was fed through a tube but could breathe independently. She was sent home as nothing more could be done in the hospital. She remained in semi-coma for 3 months until I was contacted. After 3 weeks of the treatment, she regained her consciousness after which further physical rehabilitation was carried out to make her walk. The TV interview showed her in perfectly normal condition.

## Coma after head-on collision on the road

A nun from the Brahma Kumari Organization, a well-known spiritual order, was involved in a head-on collision in Nepal. She was brought to India and hospitalized. After 3 months, she was discharged home, as her consciousness did not return. She was sent to their center in west Delhi where I examined her and decided to treat. An assistant was designated to treat her daily. Some 4 weeks later, she regained consciousness but was still severely disabled due to various neurological injuries. Her first words were 'Om Shanti' the popular words used by Brahma-Kumaris to greet each other.

## Coma after chocking

Another very interesting case of note was in Muscat, The Sultanate of Oman. The spiritual leader of a prominent tribe was driving home. He ate a piece of dry bread and choked. He collapsed in the car. His driver had the presence of mind to take him straight to the Royal Hospital, which was only a few minutes away. The excellent medical team resuscitated him and got his heart beating again. He was on a life support machine, as he could not breathe independently.

Two months passed but there were no further signs of consciousness. The doctors had no hope of reviving him, especially as he was 90 years old.

I was called in from London as a last hope. Hundreds of Omani people dressed in astonishingly white robes stood outside the Royal Hospital and hoped for the best for their leader. It was quite an amazing sight.

I was taken to the Intensive Care Unit where I examined him. The team of doctors explained there was nothing that they could do and given his age and state, there was no hope for him. I explained my technique and said perhaps the improved blood flow through the vertebral arteries to the brain stem; where the vital centers of respiration and heart beat are located, might just kick start the process of independent breathing. They had no clue as to what I was talking about because there was no reason for the blood to be obstructed in the vertebro-basilar arterial network. I explained that perhaps he hurt his neck when he collapsed in the car, as there was very little space available for him to fall. They were very nervous but took a written agreement from relatives and allowed me to treat him.

I treated his neck in the ICU. A couple of days later one of my brothers, Firdous trained in the technique was flown in from Delhi to continue the treatment in the Royal Hospital in Muscat.

A month later he regained consciousness but spoke very little. The entire tribe rejoiced and the medical team was very surprised. He became very quiet in his 'second life' but he was conscious, ate normally and chanted prayers. He went on to live for a couple of years more.

# Chapter 11 – Complications of Birth Injuries

## Birth injuries are becoming more common due to a variety of factors.

Women do not prepare themselves for labour, especially if they work until the last trimester. Socially, maternity leave is considered to be 'a sign of difference' from men and working women do not have much time for exercises, diet, relaxation and etc.

If the birth canal is not ready or properly relaxed and the labour contractions are weak, the head is stuck at the entrance of the neck of the uterus for a long time. With each contraction the fragile neck of the baby is put under tremendous pressure. This is what happens in prolonged (over 15 hours) of labour.

If the contractions on the other hand are vigorous, the baby's head opens up the tightened canal with great pressure and it comes out in brief but rapid labour. This is what I call the 'champagne cork' birth. The head simply 'pops' out in less than 2 hours of labour. In this case too, injuries to the neck are likely. The newborn baby is very fragile, so it can't even support the neck / head. Can you imagine the trauma it goes through with such abnormal labour?

Forceps and Ventouse delivery cause the worse trauma to the head and neck a newborn can face. The experienced hands of a qualified midwife could deliver babies perfectly. With the advance of medicine, the art has been replaced by technology. Stimulation, Suction, Caesarean operations are becoming common.

The umbilical cord around the neck can strangulate the baby. The cord is coiled around the neck and the labour force pushes the baby out. The cord is of limited length so it squeezes the neck as the baby comes out of the birth canal. If the labour is long then the trauma is intense, the baby is often born blue indicating severe lack of blood in the head. Depending on the severity and length of time the blood supply to the delicate brain is cut off, the damage to the baby's physical, emotional and physiological development also varies.

Handling the baby after birth is also very important. You have to be extremely careful with the heavy head and a floppy neck and you simply can't hold the baby with one hand and do something with the other. You open the neck area to chance trauma especially as all the muscles and vertebrae are not fully developed.

So many babies are born premature nowadays and so handling them is a delicate issue. Even though they lie flat in the incubator, they are moved, fed, changed, turned etc and these do affect the delicate neck and head area.

I can list a few of such complications that I observed in my years of practice.

# 1. Cerebral Palsy or Spasticity in the body after birth injury

This is a severe form of brain damage caused by strangulation of the two pairs of arteries supplying blood to the brain. Prolonged deprivation of blood to the brain is the primary cause of this devastating disease. It is often undiagnosed until a few months later when the child does not move the limbs or develops spasticity.

If the blood flow is reduced, for example due to the cord around the neck for 5-10 minutes during labour, the damage can be very severe. There is loss of co-ordination of movement, spasticity in the limbs and the neck, loss of speech, learning difficulties etc some children show signs of high intelligence even if they cannot walk or move their hands in co-ordination. They can't move but the brain becomes sharp as if physical energy is diverted to intellectual energy.

Upon interview, I found that the vast majority of them had cord around their neck, were born premature or had forceps delivery or some trauma sustained at labour. Some may have some genetic predisposition but that does not convince me.

## Cerebral Palsy after being born with the cord around the neck

The son of a Delhi industrialist was born with a cord around his neck and was a blue baby. After a few months the mother noticed that he didn't move much. When Cerebral Palsy was diagnosed, the family was devastated. When he was one year old, their family's yoga therapist, Swami Ram Lakhan, began to massage him for an hour a day. His neck, arms, legs, spine, head and feet were massaged with mustard oil. His movements became co-ordinated and he began to crawl, stand and walk. I was introduced to him when he was about 6 years old. He walked with his heels raised, the coordination of his hands were not perfect. He had a squint and could not speak coherently.

I began to treat his neck and massaged his legs and arms. The yoga master's treatment combined with mine began to show better results. He could run and speak better and he went to a normal school. The yoga master used his exercise techniques for coordination and movement while I focused mainly on my massage technique. This went on for several years and I bonded with the boy very well and he used to ask me a lot of questions. I left India but did see him occasionally during my trips there. Years later, I met him in his office where he was the managing director of his own company and he was married to a lovely lady. I was so pleased for him as early treatment helped him to lead a normal life.

I always believed in one simple logic: If a lack of blood flow to the brain is the primary cause of such disability, then improved circulation to the brain, at an early stage will cure it or reinstate some basic functions at least in severe ceases.

## Multiple complications after being born with a cord around the neck

An English girl was born with a cord around her neck. Her mother brought her to see me when she was 18. She regularly wet her bet, was an introvert, had poor immune system and had growth problem. I began to treat her neck every week for a year and she made steady improvements. She begun to grow, had her periods, was less tired, and stopped wetting her bet at night. I saw her recently after 6 years. She is now a beautiful young lady but still feels tired often depressed and can't focus on any work. I suggested that she should train under me to treat children with birth injuries. She is looking forward to that and I hope she is able to do that as I feel she should be independent.

## Sick children's camp – Dynamo Camp, Tuscany, Italy

A friend of mine, Enzo Manes, operates a well-organized camp for sick children with a charity called 'Hole in the Wall'. It's called Dynamo Camp and is based in Enzo's copper company's (KME) estate in northern Tuscany, Italy. Sick children go there for a highly enjoyable break where they can play, swim, sing, dance and have fun. The volunteers look after such children and so parents get a break.

I did a two-day seminar for parents of disabled children, teaching parents my technique of improving blood flow to the brain. After a while the children with cerebral palsies showed noticeable improvements as their spasticity improved, the drooling became less and they were a lot calmer. These children showed noticeable changes even though the treatments were applied much later. Dynamo Camp was not meant to be a treatment center and it is not licensed to do that. My over enthusiasm to treat those disabled children has caused a dilemma. The parents want to learn the technique but there are logistical problems. There are other children with cancer, leukaemia, genetic disorders etc and so neurologically affected children cannot be singled out. A wealthy Russian friend of mine, Georgy Bedjamov has promised to help such children. He already supports disabled children in Russia with financial help. I hope one day, I can take up the challenge to teach parents to treat their children with birth injuries.

## 2. Epilepsy after birth injury

Epilepsy is a disease of the brain characterized by periodic seizures when the body shakes violently. The normal treatment for such episodes or fits is drugs that suppress the electrical activity of the brain. The brain generates electrical charge, rather like the rain clouds, which are then sent down to the rest of the body through nerves to cause involuntary contractions of muscles in quick succession. This is called Grand Mal seizures. Another type Petit Mal causes absentia or when the person momentarily becomes blank, losing all communication with the outside world. It's like someone switching off completely for a few seconds.

I have successfully treated several children and a few adults with epilepsy. The results were so noticeable that some physicians contacted me to find out exactly how this treatment worked which I could only explain by using logic but Evidence-Based Medicine needs a scientific proof.

### Severe Epilepsy in a child

An Asian boy of four was brought in to see me in my clinic in London. The boy had 8-12 seizures a day and was put on anti-epileptic drugs. His doctor had increased the dose to the maximum but even that didn't stop the seizures. I taught the parents how to do the treatment daily at home and one of my assistants saw him at the clinic once a week. After just a few weeks, the fits stopped. He is now over eight years old and has not had any more seizures. The doctors thought they had hit the right level of drugs and were reluctant to reduce the dose but the parents stopped the medication on their own for a couple of years.

### Epilepsy after forceps delivery

When I was doing my seminar at The Dynamo Club in Tuscany, a little boy of two was brought to me. The parents were very distraught as the child had several seizures in an hour, which could not be controlled with drugs. He was a forceps delivery and was a blue baby at birth. I explained my technique, on a one to one consultation and taught both parents how to do the neck massage.

The parents did this therapy twice a day and after 3 weeks the results were astonishing as the boy had only a couple episodes a day. At the open day at The Dynamo Camp, this boy's success story was mentioned in a gathering of over a thousand parents, donors and volunteers many of whom had tears in their eyes. I am confident that he, like the others, will show good results and even get cured.

## Epilepsy in a child caused by excessive indulgence in electronic games

There was the case of an Arab child, 5 years of age who started getting fits quite suddenly. He was brought to London and had every possible test done but nothing concrete showed up in them. I examined him and asked if he played exciting video games with flashing lights. The answer was `yes'. The parents were reluctant to start any drug treatment as they were looking for some homeopathic or herbal solution to the child's problem. I managed to convince them to have a few sessions with me and also taught their nanny how to do the treatment at home. Within a few days the fits stopped and threw away all the video games.

## Epileptic fits after birth injury, leading to an emotional disorder

The son of a well-known golfer who is an old friend had up to 5 seizures in an hour. His birth was difficult as he came out with the Occiput first. His illness caused great tension in the family and the father's performance was affected by it. After two months of my treatment the seizures stopped. Sadly he then had some other emotional problem. The family moved abroad and I could not continue with his treatment, but I meet the parents at The Dunhill Golf Links Championship in St. Andrews, Scotland every year and I am pleased to know that the boy is making a steady progress.

# 3. Problem of the Immune System

The Hypothalamus-Pituitary complex must definitely give command to control the immune system. Exactly how that is done is not known but some sort of coordination has to take place. Since scientists do not know why the body suddenly produces white blood cells (our lymphocytes) in response to an invasion by bacteria in the body, they regard this as a 'spontaneous' reaction. It simply can't be so as there has to be a higher command from the brain, which has the information of everything that goes on in the body. The white blood cells behave as if they are 'individual' soldiers carrying out the job of ridding the body of the invading bacteria, virus, fungi, pollen, allergens; chemicals etc even soldiers need some High Command to coordinate their action. The number and type of white blood cells and where they should be directed, depends on the assessment and response on the analysis of the hypothalamic-pituitary complex or axis.

## Born with a mass (Terratoma) in the lungs and persistent infection

Catherine, a three-year-old girl was brought to me with a very complicated history. She was born with a terratoma in the lungs. Terratoma is not a tumor but an actual foetus that doesn't grow outside the body as twin but in one of the organs of the other. It's like having a brother or sister growing inside you and not alongside, sharing the mother's blood. In this case the foetus stopped developing when it reached a tennis ball size. In a vast majority of cases, this additional foetus / twin does not differentiate much into organs and ultimately stops growing. It then becomes a 'tumour' in the body like a benign mass.

Catherine was on antibiotics ever since she was born as she coughed and was breathless all the time. Her immune system was so poor that she harboured an infection, almost continuously, in the lungs. The chances of her survival were poor.

Professor Buteyko, the well-known Russian breathing expert was my guest and staying in the flat above the clinic. He cured asthma, allergies, blood pressure etc with his retention-breath technique. It did originate in the principles of yoga but the Professor studied it for years and developed it to make it more applicable. His press interviews impressed a lot of people and we had many people calling us for appointments with him.

The mother came to see Professor Buteyko but he was very busy. When I saw her, I said I would like to treat her. Since the child was too young, she couldn't be trained to do complicated breathing exercises and so mother agreed to give me a chance.

I changed her diet and organized a daily massage using my technique. She saw me about twice a week initially for the neck and head treatment. Within weeks she started to feel better and with the cooperation of her Pediatrician I got her off antibiotics. If she had the slightest cold, she would be brought to see me and I would give her my sinus oil, extra boost of vitamins and do my trademark neck massages. Within a couple of days she would recover. Therefore, she never had antibiotics after that.

As soon as her infection was better, she, like the hundreds of children that I have treated, began to grow. As she grew the terratoma became relatively smaller and stopped occupying a proportionately large part of the lungs. Soon it became insignificant and an inert mass. Today she is a beautiful girl, rides horses and lives a normal life.  Her case was reported in The Mail on Sunday, a popular UK newspaper.

I really can't recall how many young children I have been able to help with their immune systems. It will certainly run into hundreds. Children born with Forceps or Ventouse and with various forms of birth injuries, have in as many as 90% of cases had some complications or the other in early childhood. The most common one amongst them is frequent colds and coughs. These children will catch infections very easily. They get allergies like eczema, asthma etc as well.

# 4. Eczema and Asthma after birth injury

## Eczema after birth injury

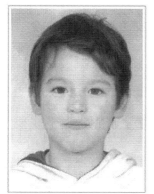

Hektor, a boy barely 10 weeks old was brought to me with exudative (oozing) eczema. The mother hardly had any milk and the baby was fed with formula milk from day one. The birth of the baby was also complicated. That was the youngest baby I had seen with such widespread eczema.

I explained to the mother that I needed her full cooperation in the baby's diet and treatment. I taught her how to massage the neck, spine and also general areas like the arms and legs. At first she was nervous but then got used to giving him massage every night before bed. I introduced solid organic food at 5 months using pureed fresh food and finally at 6 months or so, the eczema started to improve and the patches were restricted to the hands, elbows, and ankles. The treatment continued and in about 18 months he was clear of eczema. I used homeopathic remedies for any colds or coughs he had and never used antibiotics. I had an understanding with the mother that if the child had any signs of an ongoing infection like running nose, sneezing slight fever etc she would bring him to me as soon as possible. I would use massage, vitamin drops, my sinus oil drops for the nose and diet which works every time.

# Refusal for trial using my technique to treat eczema and asthma in children

In 1994, I had collected my patient's notes (some 25 of them), and with the help of my friend Dr Michael Gurmley, a well-known GP, went to see Dr Andrew Bush, a consultant at The Royal Brompton Hospital in London. I explained how by using a simple but nourishing diet, massage and breathing exercises, I was able to treat eczema and asthma in children. He was quite impressed with the explanation I gave him about the neck treatment.

Further communication was started and we spoke about setting up a trial using my technique.

After a few weeks, I got a disappointing letter from Dr Bush saying that the Ethical Committee at the hospital refused to accept the proposal to carry out this trial. The reason given was quite unspecific. They said the diet and massage weren't a treatment and so could not be used for a clinical trial.

## Born with a mass in the lung

Years later I was called by a mother to see her daughter at The Royal Brompton Hospital. She begged me to see her even though she was admitted in the Intensive Care Unit. I saw the notes and saw that the 2 year old was a patient of Professor Andrew Bush.

 The child had been born with a terratoma (see Catherine's case earlier in this chapter) in the liver and the large mass pushed the diaphragm up. This caused constant breathlessness so she had a Tracheotomy (a tube in her bronchus) for artificial breathing. She was on antibiotics from the day she was born as she had constant chest infection. She was fed via a tube so I recommended marrowbone soup, vitamins and mineral drops and taught the mother to do the neck massage. I also sent a colleague to do the treatment in the hospital once a week.

After two months, when her breathing was stable, she was taken off antibiotics and discharged home. The treatment continued at the home and the little girl began to run around and became a joy for the parents. The tracheotomy was kept open as a precaution just in case she had a lung infection but she never did.

When the little girl was about 5 years old, the doctors decided to remove the benign terratoma from the liver. It was a risky surgery that was to last several hours. The parents agreed, as they wanted their lovely daughter to lead a normal life.

I got a call late on the day of the surgery from the mother to say that her daughter died on the operation table. I was deeply saddened. If the treatment continued, she would have grown further and the tumor mass would have become proportionality small but you needed time for that.

## 5. Stimulating growth in children with neck treatment

Almost all of the children I have treated using my technique have had a spurt of growth as the pituitary gland produces more growth hormone. In fact I tell the parents who do the treatment to their children that as soon as they notice growth in their children, they should know that the treatment is working well. It is a telltale sign of the hypothalamic-pituitary area being stimulated.

I often wonder why so many children are experiencing rapid growth nowadays. The population in general is taller now in the developed countries than in the past. It must either be something in the diet that is stimulating the growth hormone or that the pituitary gland is functioning abnormally in response to the increased stress around the children.

## 6. Psychological or emotional problems in children with history of birth injury

Children born with birth injuries or have trauma to the head and neck area, often have emotional problems. These children often become hyperactive, fidgety, break things in the house, become very demanding, show signs of autism etc Most children with hyperactivity or Attention Deficit Disorder (ADD) had some sort of trauma at birth or shortly afterwards. This could be a co-incidence but an amazing one, if so. Neck massages started earlier can help such children.

### Chesty baby

The son of a friend was born with a forceps delivery. He was a slight chesty baby and as the mother was very health conscious so she tried to feed him properly. One day at dinner, I saw her son unusually hyperactive. I asked her if he had some birth trauma and she confirmed that. She also said that the teachers at the play school where he was going were complaining about him being rough with the children. She was even called to the school a couple of times for his slightly violent behaviour. This child, like most hyperactive children, demanded sweets all the time, which is an indication that the appetite center in the brain was not receiving enough glucose through the blood. I warned her that he could get further complications and so she should start the neck massage. She went down the conventional medical way, consulting pediatrician and child psychologists as it was difficult to control him and so drugs were prescribed to calm him down. Then he had his first epileptic fit and more followed. She had to go back to her country form London to take better care of him. Sadly, the boy became an autistic and now has special care.

# Conclusion

I can confirm that many children born with some degree of trauma at birth have emotional problems later as they grow. In the early stage of their life you may not notice much change as children are often naughty or very quiet but when they reach their teens, eating disorders, depression and poor self esteem often manifest themselves. Those who do sports and enjoy general well being overcome their difficulties quite well.

It is not easy to prove the link between emotional problems and birth injuries as easy as it is to prove the physical symptoms. One of the reasons is that emotional problems or behavioural problems cannot be easily quantified. There are a lot of people in society who need psychological help but get on with life because they themselves do not complain or see it as a problem. It's others who suffer because of their behaviour. So nobody can do anything about it unless his or her behaviour becomes criminal or totally unacceptable.

# Chapter 12 – Nervous Disorders

## Cranial Nerves

Cranial nerves are those that originate in the brain while all other nerves originate in the spinal cord. There are 12 pairs of cranial nerves that emerge from the skull or cranium. As they have direct links with the brain, circulatory deficiency to their centres in the subconscious brain or their roots (as they emerge from the brain) will cause corresponding malfunction of these nerves.

All nerves need nourishment, as they are physiologically very active. The nerves and their roots have very tiny capillaries called vasa nervosum (blood vessels of the nerves).

In post-trauma, as in whiplash injury, a lot of people suffer from visionary problems like partial loss of vision, blurred vision, double vision, tinnitus, facial pain, loss of sense of smell, loss of taste etc these symptoms may not be noticed immediately after the accident but can manifest later. It is for this delayed effect, that there is often a big dispute between the insurance companies and the claimants. In the UK the number of claims from whiplash injuries has risen by 18% in recent years.

## 1. Half-sided pain on the face (Trigeminal Neuralgia)

This is often called 'Tic Dolores' or episodic painful attacks on the face. If you consider all the pains in the body, then kidney stones will take the number one position followed by Migraine and Trigeminal Neuralgia. It is so painful that one should not wish this pain or your worst enemy. During an attack, one half side of the face will hurt intensely.

### House-bound for 8 years because of facial pain

A 75-year lady from Melbourne, Australia was house-bound for 8 years because of the facial pain due to Neuralgia of the top and middle branch of the Trigeminal nerve. She had a face-lift and the skin was straightened with a cut to the front of the ear, where the Trigeminal nerve emerges out of the skull. The nerve got inflamed due to a trauma caused during surgery or perhaps got compressed by the formation of scar tissue.

Her pain was so severe that the slightest touch would trigger off the attack, which would last for several minutes or hours. She couldn't wash her face or hair or apply cream or care for her face. She never went out, as she felt unclean and slept only on good side. She avoided draught on her face, as even this would trigger the attack and so she used to wear a scarf on her face all the time.

She heard of me from a mutual friend and called me and I promised to do my best. She was too afraid to fly as she was petrified of the aircraft's air conditioning.

After several months of postponement, she finally flew to London with her 85-year partner. She had severe pain and terrible jet lag when she arrived so she rested in her hotel. Finally after two days she came to see me in the clinic and was very nervous as she thought I would touch or massage the area that was affected. She was totally surprised when I treated her neck. She was greatly relieved even after the first treatment and then she became confident.

After only 5 sessions, the pain disappeared and she was euphoric. She went to the hairdressers, had facials and even dyed her hair for the first time in 8 years. She began to smile again; even smiling could trigger the attack in the past. It changed her entire life. She had massage from my assistant who had moved to Australia and so could continue her treatment.

## Conference on Trigeminal Neuralgia

In 1996, I was invited to speak at a conference on Trigeminal Neuralgia where dentists discussed various causes of the disease. Most seem to think that the artery (a branch of the vertebro-basilar artery) that feeds the Trigeminal nerve makes a loop around it and mechanically scratches or irritates it, causing severe pain. In 30% of cases, scans show that this artery does have anomalies or loops. My argument was: what happens in the other 70% of cases? I made a confident and convincing presentation, explaining my stand on the reduced blood supply to the Trigeminal nerve, as the main cause. The dentists were impressed and found the logical explanation very convincing. They were not so appreciative when I added that during excessive dental work, the neck is often traumatized as the vertebrae get disaligned and this often causes Trigeminal Neuralgia. I should have been more diplomatic as they have to do whatever they have to do. They are not to blame. They probably need to operate with special chairs or with patients lying flat or under general anaesthesia in complicated cases. The problem is that they have to work the jaws and thus the neck gets affected in few cases.

## Facial pain for six years

A Spanish aristocrat lady came to see me in Madrid. She was petrified of touching her face. For six years, life for her was hell because of the one-sided facial pain, which was constant. On questioning it was clear that she had had some accidents. I treated her neck and after the first session she felt relief so I gave her a few more sessions and she was pain free. She couldn't believe it as she thought she would have to live with it.

# 2. Loss of Taste and Smell

After whiplash injuries, head injuries and other traumas in that area many people experience loss of taste or smell. Since these sensory functions are not lost immediately after the trauma but manifest themselves months later, it is difficult to link the symptoms to the cause.

These Cranial nerves are highly sensitive and delicate nerves so improving blood flow after a long gap doesn't always help. One doesn't know the damage until much later so treatments cannot be applied in time. I have a few cases where treatment was applied within weeks of the loss of sense of smell and the results were good.

## Loss of sense of smell after a fall

A young man in his late 20'tripped and fell on his face. Immediately the sense of smell was lost but a few months later he started smelling coffee all the time. I gave him a session of neck therapy and gave him some aromatherapy oil to smell. He was surprised that he could smell again so I told him to continue with neck massage with a sports injury therapist. I met him a few months later and he said that he could smell a lot better.

# 3. Loss of Vision

The optic nerve that is responsible for vision is located close to the pituitary gland. The same circle of arteries that feed it, also supply nutrition to the Optic nerves. Whether your hearing, taste and smell has improved or deteriorated slightly is hard to tell, but if your vision has changed you will notice it immediately. Most people who have neck manipulation and almost everyone who has my treatment of the neck, report sudden and amazing brightness in the eyes. They say that they can see well as more blood flows into the Optic nerve. It may not be a permanent after just one treatment, as it will take a few sessions to achieve long-term results.

## An airline pilot's partial loss of field vision in one eye

A 747 pilot of Cathay Pacific was climbing a hill in Hong Kong when he fell and hit his head on the rock. He was airlifted to a hospital in an unconscious state. Later he had headaches, dizziness, fatigue, and partial loss of field vision on one side. It was this last symptom which worried him the most because as a pilot he had to have perfect vision. He came to see me in my clinic in Hong Kong and I began to treat his neck and gave him some yogic eye exercises. His vision began to improve after a few sessions so he joined me on my Himalayan Health Trip, where the effect of altitude and massage further improved the blood supply to the nerve. The combined effort of raised haemoglobin and treatment with my technique helped him tremendously. He went back for an eye test, had a few extra training sessions at the simulator and went back to flying again.

## Loss field vision in one eye

Some 20 years ago, a close friend of mine, Frank Chapman, lost vision on one-half of the field in one eye, after a fall. He was extremely worried as driving, reading, working became very difficult. He went to the best doctors in London and steroids were prescribed but that didn't help at all. I showed him the yogic eye exercises and began to treat his neck area. After only a few sessions his eyesight improved and the field of vision was restored to normal. Since then we have remained close family friends.

## Partial loss of vision after a fall

A gamekeeper came to see me for partial loss of vision and had to retire because of his eye condition. I asked him if he had any head or neck injury. Initially he said he didn't but midway through my treatment he said he had fallen off a horse and hit his head on a rock. Shortly after that his vision started to deteriorate. The link was thus established. He had some treatments and I showed his wife how to massage the neck and he also did the eye exercises, which is my standard treatment for all eye problems. His vision was restored to normal and he was back to work.

## Partial loss of vision in one eye after a neck injury

The owner of a large Estate in Scotland had partial loss of vision in one eye. He came to see me after recommendation from a friend. I asked him about any accident he may have had prior to the onset of this symptom but he could not recall any accident or trauma ever. He came back the following day and said he recalled an incident prior to the visionary problems. He was carrying the gun over his shoulders and had both his arms on either side of the gun and as he walked, he felt dizzy and slightly sick. He sat down immediately to rest. He felt better but a few days later his vision started to deteriorate. He was quite amazed at the link between the neck trauma and his symptom, as he had never thought of it.

Very often people can't recall physical accidents but after the treatment, the improved blood flow stimulates the memory center in the limbic system of the brain and patients are able to recall better.

People who are about to faint see darkness but if they are helped immediately to lie horizontally, the vision is restored as blood flows into the retina and optic nerve. This is a direst proof that lack of blood in the optic nerves causes loss of vision.

# 4. Hypothalamic-Pituitary malfunction

Both the pituitary gland and the hypothalamus get blood supply from a ring of arteries called 'The Circle of Willis', a major branch of the vertebro-basilar arteries. Impaired blood flow to this vital area of the brain can cause serious health problem.

## a. Thyroid Malfunction

The thyroid glands are located in front of the neck. Iodine absorbed in the gut is transported to the thyroid glands where the cells manufacture and release the thyroid hormones. Both the synthesis and secretion of thyroid hormones are controlled by the pituitary hormone called the thyroid-stimulating hormone (TSH). So if the body needs more thyroid hormones the hypothalamus, sensing the deficiency, will signal the pituitary gland to secrete TSH, kick start the manufacturing process and release it. Thus there is a strong link between the headquarters and the factory.

Functions of thyroid hormones are quite simple. These hormones penetrate all cells of the body and help to generate energy. They facilitate "burning" of glucose and thus increase the metabolic rate. The more glucose you burn the more energy you get. If thyroid secretion is less, the metabolic rate drops, the body slows down. The excess glucose, which is available through digestion, will then get deposited as fat and patients will experience weight gain, cold hands and feet, feel hot and cold, hair loss, low blood pressure, depression, dry skin, constipation and chronic fatigue. The normal solution is to prescribe Thyroxin, the synthetic thyroid hormone, which helps with fatigue, low blood pressure, abnormal heat sensation etc but does not change the weight. That is because the fat deposited all over the body is hormonal white cellulite fat and not dietary yellow fat, which "burns off" very easily. People did not eat extra to gain this weight, as it is just that there was a fault that resulted in the reduction of the metabolic rate.

There are other causes of thyroid malfunction. Lack of iodine in diet causes poor synthesis of thyroid hormones. The TSH makes the gland swell up but the thyroid hormones secretion is poor. The large swelling of thyroid gland is called goiter.

Excessive production of thyroid hormones which is a "panic state" of Hypothalamic-Pituitary complex, causes muscular tension, increased metabolism, flushing, excessive body heat, increased heart rate, panic attacks, anxiety, restlessness, mood swings, excessive sweating and weight loss. Despite the increased activity of the thyroid the body feels totally exhausted. The person feels as if he or she has run a marathon.

Most people, who suffer from Hypothalamic-Pituitary malfunction, have a history of birth injuries, trauma, accidents, whiplashes, neck injuries etc Thyroid malfunction is often directly linked to that.

### b.  Disturbances in Periods (Menstruation)

The Pituitary stimulates the ovaries through the hormone Follicle Stimulating Hormone (FSH). This causes the maturation of the follicles that ultimately cause ovulation. Being the headquarters of the autonomous or subconscious functions of the body, the hypothalamus, together with the pituitary, controls the menstrual cycle.

## Lack of periods for 6 months after old head and neck trauma

A young lady did not have periods for over 6 months. She tried the pill but that didn't help. Her specialists told her that she was menopausal and really depressed her. She came to see me and I asked her about any accident she may have had. She confirmed she fell down the stairs as a child, hit her head a couple of times and cut her chin in childhood. I explained what the problem was and I changed her diet, gave her some supplements and gave her a series of neck treatment. After two months she was ecstatic as she got her first period after a long time. She had slight irregular periods for 6 months and then they became regular.

I have numerous cases of women who came to see me with period disturbances of various types. Some had long or frequent periods; some had very brief (2 days) and scanty periods while others had long cycles (over 35 days). The treatment that helped them was my technique of neck and shoulder massage.

### c.  Infertility

There are many women who, in spite of having normal periods and whose husbands / partners have perfect sperm count, fail to get pregnant. Such women are extremely stressed and IVF and other artificial methods of conception often fail. Relatives, friends and colleagues often ask why they do not want to start a family. A woman feels incomplete with infertility.

I have my own explanation for this. Stress does play an important role. The blood supply to the endometrium or innermost layer of the uterus is provided by vessels that penetrate the layer of muscles horizontally. With stress the muscles contract and the blood vessels are compressed. The endometrium is starved of nutrients and the implanted fertilized egg fails to develop. Soon after ovulation, if a woman receives the sperms, the fertilization is almost guaranteed. Unfortunately if she begins to worry (will it happen or will it not). The uterus began to contract. Ultrasonic examination after a pinprick test shows that the uterus can contract involuntarily due to painful stimulus so it must do the same when in stress.

My approach is to apply various types of therapies simultaneously to achieve the results. I change the diet so there is less intake of acid foods, alcohol, coffee, excess salt and yeast (to avoid bloating in the stomach.) and increase their protein intake. The neck treatment helps the ovulation, reduces stress and creates the 'feel good factor' and yoga helps to calm the mind. Some herbal supplements are used to help to thicken the lining of the womb. This integrated approach prepares the woman's mind and body to conceive. The Daily Mail in the UK interviewed a few ladies that had babies after my treatments. One French lady had a baby after 8 years of trying and after the first one she went on to have two more with changes of diet and some neck treatments. This article brought hundreds of infertile women to my clinic but I could not accept all of them as many were in their forties.

## Infertility after an old accident

A woman in her late thirties tried for a child for 8 years. She had many tests, tried IVF, Chinese Medicine, Acupuncture but nothing helped. She came to see me as a last resort. She confirmed she had a bad accident when she was in her twenties and used computers a lot. I changed her diet and began to give her treatment for the neck, which was very stiff. After a couple of months, she didn't have periods and so she was worried that the treatment didn't work. The she went to her regular doctor who carried out a blood test and a scan which showed that she was pregnant. She had a lovely baby girl. Three years later, she tried for a second child but nothing happened so she came back to see me and I recommended the same treatment. The following month she became pregnant and this time she had a son. This lady jokingly called them Dr Ali's children. From time to time I see the children for some minor ailments.

## Married for seven years without children

My friends Sophie and Thomas who lived in London were married for seven years. They could not have children. I invited them to go to the Himalayas with me to relax and have all the treatments (yoga, massage, walks and meditation). We had a wonderful time together. A few months after we came back, Sophie called me to say she was pregnant. They move to Munich and now they have two more children.

### d.  Hormonal Imbalances in Children after birth injuries

## Six year girl with hormonal imbalances

A six year old Sikh girl was brought to see me by her parents in London. They were absolutely horrified that their daughter developed breasts, had pubic hair and began to spot regularly as if she had periods. They went to the specialists who recommended drugs that blocked hormones, which meant she would be infertile forever.

The girl was a forceps delivery and was blue at birth. I had never seen such a case before so I thought may be stimulating the pituitary might kick-start the self-regulatory system of the body. I gave her some diet and taught the parents my massage technique. Within three months the treatment started to work. The pubic hair gradually disappeared and there was no spotting of blood. They continued the treatment for a year but breast however, did not regress. Today she is a beautiful 26 years old with full signs of femininity. That case convinced me in my mind that hormonal problems can be treated with my method if patients fully comply with the recommendations.

## Strong body odour due to hormonal imbalance in a child

The grand daughter of a well-known businessman in London was 6 years old when the mother noticed that she was developing breasts. Additionally, she developed strong body odour. No child would go near her in school and so she developed a complex. The school complained and specialists were at their wits end as they just first didn't know what to do.

My brother, Imran, began to treat her at the clinic once a week while the nanny and the mother did some more treatment at home. After a few months the breasts stopped developing and the body odour was less intense. She began to grow with the treatment and so the breast did not look very prominent

Male goats have a very distinct smell and one can identify them from afar. Similarly, children with severe hormonal problems have a strong body odour. I wish I had seen more cases to study the changes before, during and after treatments but such cases are rare.

## e. Polycystic Ovarian Syndrome (PCOS)

The Hypothalamic-Pituitary complex stimulates the development of round chambers or follicles in the ovaries where egg cells grow. Every month, by around mid-cycle, one or the other follicle bursts and releases the egg cell. This process is called ovulation. Sometimes due to the over-activity of the Hypothalamic-Pituitary area, one or more of the follicles to grow abnormally large. Multiple cysts are called polycystic ovaries and the complex of symptoms that these conditions produces in the body is called Polycystic Ovarian Syndrome (PCOS).

In male and female bodies Testosterone is the principal hormone. In females, however, testosterone is converted in the ovaries into Estrogen. Due to the presence of cysts in the ovaries, the healthy tissue is displaced and the above conversion is not possible. Thus in PCOS, there is an excess of testosterone or male hormones in the body as a result of which the periods stop or become erratic and these women get facial hair, acne and put on excess weight (cellulite fat).

I have seen many patients with this condition. They are usually young, in their 20s and 30s. Some were infertile because of erratic or absence of periods. Initially I suggest a fat-free diet which over a period of time forces the body to break down its own fat. An exercise programme enhances this weight loss. Amazingly, just the weight loss alone can trigger the recovery from PCOS in some women.

I integrate the weight-loss programme with neck treatment (at least twice a month), phyto-estrogens (Don Quai or Shatavari), Homeopathic remedies (Pulsatilla where indicated) and some vitamins and minerals. In a majority of cases this treatment works and the cysts reduce in size or disappear. The facial hair disappears only when everything else is rectified. In PCOS, the insulin level is often raised and so many women are prescribed Metformin, an anti-diabetic drug. My integrated approach to treatment of PCOS diminishes the need for this drug especially when the weight drops with diet control.

### f.  Auto-Immune Diseases

In auto-immune diseases something strange happens. Normally, all tissues of the body are very friendly even though they have different cells carrying out different functions as they have the same parents (egg and sperm) and are related: no problem there. Sometimes, due to infections, inflammation or some unknown factors, some tissues are so deeply affected that their genetic structure or identity code is changed. Such tissues include joint membrane, skin, kidneys, eyes, thyroid, muscles, gut lining, blood vessels etc The immune system identifies them instantly as 'traitors' or aliens and begins to attack these tissues. That is a bizarre reaction as the body tries to destroy or reject its own tissue, as if a tissue transplant has really gone wrong.

The angry immune system becomes more intolerant and the only way physicians can stop it is by prescribing immuno-suppressants like methotrexate, steroids etc by suppressing the immune system you spare the affected tissues from being totally destroyed with serious consequences.

Since the Hypothalamic-Pituitary Complex controls all involuntary functions, I presumed that helping it to function better would in some way help to check this aggressive disease and to my great satisfaction, it worked in many cases. If patients with auto-immune disease changed their lifestyle, controlled their stress and received my specific neck treatment, there was a good chance that the disease would go into remission. I call it 'remission' because these diseases are nasty and with more stress and bad lifestyle, they can return with a vengeance.

### g.  Chilblains and Reynaud's Syndrome

These are autoimmune diseases that affect smaller blood vessels of the hands and feet. The circulation is severely impaired .

## Severe Chilblains

Sister Stella, the principal of Convent of Jesus and Mary in Delhi, India, suffered from severe Chilblains; even in the summer her toes would ulcerate and become purple. She couldn't wear shoes and had difficulty in standing or walking. She wore woollen socks, dipped her feet in warm saline water, used a hot water bottle under her feet at bedtime and dressed the ulcers when they appeared.

Frankly speaking, it was a challenging case for me. However, I recommended a general treatment of diet, simple yoga, some supplements and weekly neck treatment. To my great relief she began to respond. She had comfortable summers and had fewer problems in the winters. I was in touch with her for a while. She was quite pleased with the results and had regular neck treatments. Sadly, she died after a few years.

## Freezing white hands after washing in cold water

A leading designer in London had Reynaud's Syndrome. Her hands would go white from the wrists downwards every time she washed her hands in cold water. It looked as if she wore white gloves. The cold water would cause the arteries in the hands to constrict such that there would be a total shut down of blood flow and the hands would be ice cold and painful as if she was holding ice. It was embarrassing too as those who were near would be horrified to see 'white' hands.

A mutual friend, Stephen Marks sent her to see me. I explained what was happening and because it was freshly diagnosed there was a good chance that it would heal. She followed the treatment religiously and after washing her hands she would practice my special breathing. I asked her to hold her breath for 10 seconds, take in only half a breath and hold it again for 10 seconds. Effectively speaking, she was taking 3-4 breaths in a minute instead of the 16 or so that we normally take. This causes raised carbon dioxide in blood, alarming the Hypothalamus of an eminent danger of oxygen deprivation. The hypothalamus in turn would send messages to the arteries in the hands to dilate instantly. This counteracted the effect of the Reynaud's syndrome. She was thrilled that the neck massage and breathing technique worked and saw me regularly for 3 months. She never had the attack again and began to feel overall quite well.

### h. Rheumatoid Arthritis

This chronic inflammatory disease attacks both smaller and larger joints of the body. There is swelling, pain, restricted movement and severe morning stiffness. Nowadays, doctors go straight for steroids and immuno-suppressants to calm down the symptoms. It is considered to be an incurable disease that affects mostly women.

## Acute Rheumatoid Arthritis

Cecilia an old friend was totally distraught when she was diagnosed with Rheumatoid Arthritis. The early morning stiffness and the pain were unbearable but she was very reluctant to take those heavy drugs.

At the first meeting, I told her that if she did what I suggested, the chances were that she would go into a long remission. She had old childhood traumas but her neck was stiff due to a lot of stress for a prolonged period.

I changed her diet and did a 7 day course of treatment of the neck and some of the joints that were severely affected. I used my well-known Joint Oil that contained a blend of mustard, sesame, clove, winter green and black cumin seed oil. She massaged her joints every night at bed-time. This oil helped to reduce the pain and inflammation in the joints.

After a week she started to feel better but continue to have massage therapy form a local therapist. After 6 months all her pain and inflammation disappeared. A blood test showed reduction of ESR, an indicator of inflammation in the body. Four years later, when I last saw her, she was totally asymptomatic. She recommended one other friend with a similar condition, and she too is making good progress. Her husband Jan was so pleased with her progress that he made a substantial donation to my Sagoor Charity Clinic in the Himalayas. A guest-house was built there for foreign patients to have treatments for chronic ailments at an affordable price. The guest-house now helps to fund medicines for the 50000 or so people who use it. It was a great help to them.

## Chronic Rheumatoid Arthritis

An elderly lady from a very well-known Aristocratic family in Florence had severe Rheumatoid Arthritis. It restricted her movement and deeply affected her social life. She came to see me at The Castel Monastero near Siena in Italy where she had the neck treatment periodically and that completely changed her life. She has treatment of the neck from time to time for her tinnitus, dizziness and fatigue which are all part of The Ali Syndrome.

### i.   Psoriasis (Skin disease)

This is one of the most difficult skin conditions to treat. It affects the elbows, knees, scalp, face, body, soles of the feet, hands etc Very often it is linked to stress but it is an autoimmune disease. Normal treatment involves steroid creams and immune-suppressants, people often get the skin cured in the Dead Sea or in hyper-saline water used in Thalassotherapy. The hyper-saline solution and the sun give temporary relief to the skin, but the condition returns after a few weeks when people return to their normal life.

Just as with the other autoimmune diseases, the sooner the treatment is applied the better it is.

## Psoriasis after neck injuries

A man in his forties had had several accidents from motorbike to skiing. He went through a difficult divorce and was extremely stressed. He started getting dry patches on the elbows, knees and the body. The affected area would often ooze when the dry white skin peeled off and at night there would be a lot of itching. He used coal tar, steroid creams, ultra-violet radiation etc which gave him temporary relief.

I put him on a diet of no yeast, sugar, alcohol, mushrooms, citric fruits, coffee etc I prescribed my Detox Powder, to control the yeast or Candida overgrowth in the gut. I gave him sulphur powder mixed in coconut oil which he applied on the affected areas of the skin and he had weekly neck massage.

After a few weeks the skin began to clear up. New spots would appear elsewhere but as time went by they would be smaller in size. After about 4 months his skin cleared up. He continued the treatment for about 6 months and he was cured.

### j.   Lupus (a sever autoimmune disease)

This is a debilitating autoimmune disease which attacks multiple organs like joints, kidneys, eyes, skin. Its characteristic sign is the red butterfly on the cheeks, formed by two bright red patches on both cheeks (wings) and the red nose (body). Special blood tests help in diagnosis of this condition.

## Diagnosed with Lupus

A young lady who was diagnosed with Lupus came to see me within 6 months of the tests. She had had injuries from birth and had a car accident. She suffered from backache for many years but it was when her eyes and her gait were affected, that she went to the doctors.

I gave her some neck treatment and recommended few back and eye exercises. Her eyesight gradually improved and she could walk more comfortably. The tests however did not show much change but the treatment brought her condition into remission.

I wrote a column for The Mail on Sunday in the UK for almost 6 years. I used to answer reader's questions every week. Once I wrote about my treatment for Lupus. A patient who had had treatment for this condition from me and went into remission, had difficulty in convincing her professor, who had treated her for a while that my treatment worked. She took the article to him, thinking that he would be convinced that sometimes 'Alternative' treatments worked on chronic diseases. The professor wrote to me to stop making claims and confusing patients about treatment of Lupus. There is no cure for this condition, he wrote, and it remains a life-threatening disease. I face such criticism from time to time but it doesn't stop me from doing what I do.

### k.  Premature Menopause

A lot of women, who have had serious accidents or head injuries, often begin their menopause around 40. They may not have any symptoms like irregular periods or hot flushes, but generally the periods would suddenly stop. If they have had children, they do not panic much and accept it as an unfortunate thing and get on with life. Sometimes, extreme stress can bring out this condition too. Once the menopause sets in, it is difficult to reverse it so the sooner the treatment is applied, the better the results.

## Periods stopped at 42

I did have a patient, however, who came to see me when her periods had stopped at 42 years, for only 6 months. This is often referred to as secondary amenorrhoea. She had had a whiplash injury after which she suffered from headaches and dizziness for quite sometime.

I changed her diet, put her on natural phytoestrogens, Mexican Yam, homeopathic remedies and gave her weekly neck massages. The periods came back after 3 months and became more or less regular. She had her natural menopause at 48 years.

## Menopause at 40

A lady from Alma Ata, Kazakhstan, had a bad car accident in her 30s when she lost consciousness for a while. Her life changed after that as she was anxious, irritable, had constant fatigue, memory loss and had menopause when she was 40 and continued to feel miserable. She came to see me for chronic fatigue, insomnia and aches and pains. I changed her diet and recommended the neck treatment. After 6-7 months, as she felt better and she started to have irregular but scanty periods. Her doctors were worried and so they investigated her for cancer as they suspected that the bleeding was due to malignancy. It was the natural return of periods and there was no other cause.

There are many examples of the neck treatment being beneficial for secondary amenorrhea. Many such women have had hormone therapy but the neck treatment is the most natural way of treating them.

### 1.   Food intolerances and skin allergies

As I mentioned before, the Hypothalamic-Pituitary region regulates the immune system. Food intolerances or skin allergies are local reaction of the skin or gut due to unwanted particles on those surfaces (either gut lining or skin).

Let's say you are allergic to soap, powder or a cream. Shortly after these chemicals come into contact with the skin, there will be a rash or an allergic reaction. Similarly if you are intolerant to chillies or fungal cheese, you will get bloating, cramps, diarrhoea etc as the gut lining will react unfavourably. Food intolerances should not be confused with food allergies, as the latter is a reaction of the entire immune system.

Children with multiple food intolerances respond to my treatment. They often get abdominal pain and bloating from cow's milk but if you change to goat or camel or soya milk the digestive problems disappear

Adult food intolerance has to be treated over a period of 4 months or so with my method as shorter periods of treatment do not produce satisfactory results. I have a belief or hypothesis that red blood cells and immune cells (lymphocytes) replace themselves in 125 days or so, which is 4 months. One has to, therefore, carry out an exclusion diet and neck massages for that length of time.

## Multiple food intolerances

A woman with multiple food intolerances (aubergines, cheese, yeast, pork, pineapple and tomatoes) came to see me. With these products she would get bloating, diarrhoea, agitation in the mind, headache and chronic fatigue. She had several accidents in childhood and was concussed after a skiing accident. I put this lady on a diet that excluded citric fruits, alcohol, coffee, spicy food and sugars. She also avoided the foodstuffs that she was intolerant for four months. She had almost weekly massage, did yoga and took my Detox Tea for her Candida. After 6 months she could eat some of the foodstuffs that she was initially intolerant to. I also told her that she should not eat all the troublesome foodstuffs on the same day. She managed her intolerance extremely well after that.

## Intolerant to garlic

A dear friend of mine, Ken Bridgewater, who edited the first edition of this book, was intolerant to garlic. In a club he belonged to they used to call him "Mr No-garlic". Since meeting me he had gone on my India trips and had numerous sessions of massage and yoga. He came to lunch one day and saw me cooking chicken with garlic. He was petrified and asked me politely if I could cook something else without garlic. I didn't as I was convinced that he was cured with so many sessions of treatment. He commented that if he was going to be ill there was no place like a doctor's house. He was amazed that he didn't get any reaction at all. He now eats garlic comfortably. Ken and his lovely wife Aileen have followed my Neck Connection theory and its amazing success for over 20 years.

## m. Allergies (Hay Fever, Urticaria, Eczema)

Allergy is body's natural reaction to invading non-living particles or chemicals. For living organisms (bacteria, viruses) body's immune system develops antibodies to destroy them. Vaccinations against infectious diseases like cholera, mumps, measles, typhoid, polio, tetanus use this ability to create antibodies in the body to ward off a real infection.

Even though allergic reactions are defensive reactions, the symptoms they produce are very uncomfortable. In the case of allergies, the other reactions are watery eyes, runny nose, itchy eyes, diarrhoea, hay fever, coughs, asthma attacks (wheezing) itchy skin, hives (Urticaria) etc all of which are uncomfortable.

Allergies are difficult to treat but individuals do respond to an integrated approach using diet, massage, breathing exercises, homeopathy, desensitization with diluted allergens, natural remedies, acupuncture etc a hit and trial method of selecting the best treatment for an individual is also very helpful.

I recommend a diet of no yeast, fungus, citric; alcohol, coffee, sugar diet and they regularly have neck treatments. If they have runny nose, allergic coughs or wheezing, sneezing etc, they would be advised to do the special breathing exercises. They breathe in for 6 seconds, hold breath for 6 seconds and breathe out after 6 seconds. In this way, instead of breathing 18 times in a minute (which is normal) they breathe approximately 3 times. This type of breathing dilates the nasal passage and bronchial tract and eases the symptoms. Additionally, I recommend my

Sinus Oil or plain sesame oil drops for the nose which forms a protective layer on the nose and prevents the particles (pollen, dust, mites, pollutant) and chemicals (sprays, perfumes, paint spirits, petrol fumes) from coming in contact with the mucosa of the nasal lining. So there is reduced irritation of the nasal tract and subsequent allergic reaction.

In my experience and opinion, Candida, a fungus, thrives on the gut wall rather like mould on bread, sending raphae (roots) deep into the lining thus creating micro pores. Large gut toxins, which normally cannot penetrate the gut lining, find these pores useful in passing through the barrier to reach the underlying blood vessels. These are too large to be eliminated through the kidneys so only option is the skin and sinus.

The toxins leak out of the blood vessels of the skin that swells up and looks like orange peel (hives). As the leaked fluid contains a lot of salt, the nerve endings under the skin begin to itch violently. Thus in hives you have the sudden raised patches of skin producing unbearable itch all over the body. The only immediate solution is anti-histamine or steroid injection to stop the blood vessels from dilating and leaking fluid out.

For hives, my diet and neck treatments have been very useful for many patients with chronic hives. I also recommend my Detox Tea to curtail Candida growth in the gut. This integrated approach has helped quite a number of people.

I end this chapter on Hypothalamic-Pituitary malfunction with the case history of a friend who is well-known singer and musician in Istanbul. This beautiful lady had everything going for her until one moment when her life turned upside down. After a flight, she opened the overhead luggage compartment, when a case of whisky fell right on the top of her head. She collapsed and felt dizzy. What followed later was heart breaking as she had fibromyalgia (pain all over the body), endometriosis (painful and irregular periods), panic attacks, short-term memory loss, Mellasma (brown spots on the cheeks), headaches, dizziness, sensitivity to light, freezing hands and feet, food intolerances, severe mood swing, loss of libido, skin allergies, insomnia etc. It was her music, her determination and encouragement from friends that keep her going. She is improving under my care.

# Part - III

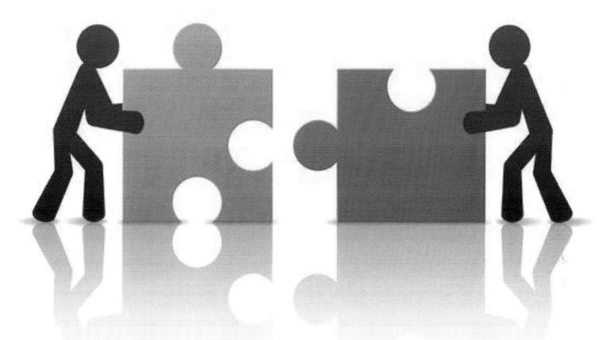

# The Solution

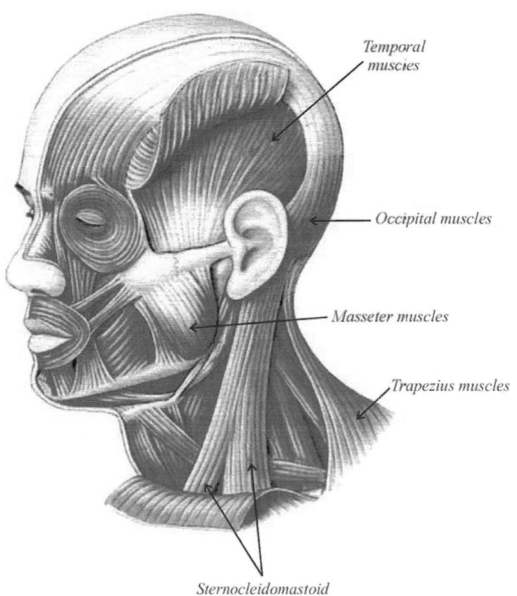

*Temporal muscles*

*Occipital muscles*

*Masseter muscles*

*Trapezius muscles*

*Sternocleidomastoid muscles*

# Chapter 13 – Historical

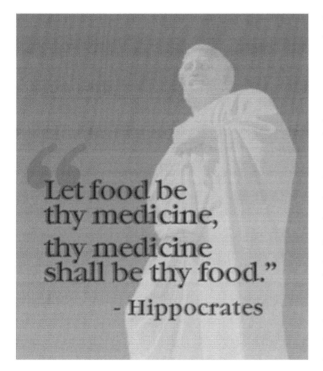

"Let food be thy medicine, thy medicine shall be thy food."
- Hippocrates

Hippocrates, who lived 2400 years ago in Greece, was regarded as the Father of Modern Medicine. His Oath is still taken by Graduating Physicians today before embarking on the practice of Medicine.

The neck is a part of a whole body and should not be treated in isolation. Indeed, its treatment has to be considered in the light of all the treatments available today. Let's start at square one. To fully appreciate the present status of medicine it is necessary to have some understanding of how it developed historically. Hippocrates, who lived 2400 years ago in Greece, was regarded as the Father of Modern Medicine. His Oath is still taken by Graduating Physicians today before embarking on the practice of Medicine. If asked, no doctor now can tell you what the Hippocratic Principal of Medicine actually was. In the 11th century another great physician Avicenna who lived in Bukhara, Uzbekistan in Central Asia but travelled in the region, used Hippocratic principles to create the foundation of what is called Unani (Unan - Eastern Greece or Ionia) Medicine. It is now practised and taught mainly in South Asia in a modified way. The original principles were largely discarded as time went by.

## Hippocrates taught the following:

1.  We have an innate healing power called "physis" (pronounced feesis) within us to maintain our health. The words "physician", "physiology", "physiotherapy", "physics" etc take their roots from it. We now understand our immune system to be part of that power that defends us.

2.  The physis is a universal force present in all living beings. It analyses what goes on outside and inside our bodies, and corrects the various functions accordingly - 24 hours a day. For example if you travel to a hot country from a cold place your physis will become very active. The change of food, climate, time zones, culture etc forces the body to adapt very quickly.

3.  Physis, if nurtured, can heal almost 80% of our illnesses and diseases. Emergency medicine, traumas, genetic disorders etc constitute the other 20% and are best treated with conventional methods.

4.  Physis can be nurtured by looking after your body and mind. This is done by eating well, exercising, relaxing, using massage, swimming, using steam or sauna, fasting periodically and sleeping adequately. In other words using common sense.

5.  Natural forms of treatments (herbs, minerals, fruits, berries etc) should be used to assist the physis to carry out its functions normally.

Although a lot of time has passed since that doctrine was established, the essence of it still remains. After the death of Hippocrates, his son-in-law and others tried to establish his sayings as "dogma" or the final word in the understanding of human health and illness. There were, however, criticisms of the School of Dogmatism and so Medicine reverted to the "free thinking" mode. Christianity came and declared that diseases were a form of punishment for sins. So God's influence on diseases became profound. You pray, take necessary measures provided by medicine and you'll get better.

In the 10th century, the great Persian physician, Avicenna, revived the Hippocratic concept.

He placed a lot of emphasis on imbalance of blood, phlegm, yellow bile and black bile the four Humours as the cause and defined the constitution of individuals with a propensity to certain diseases as the underlying factor that caused illness. The four types of constitution were Sanguine, Phlegmatic, Choleric and Melancholic. A similar approach occurred independently in China (five elements) and India (Three Doshas – Vata, Pitta and Kapha)

This Humour theory was taught in Medical schools in Europe until the 16th century. Then there was the invention of the microscope and other instruments for examination of the body. The body was viewed as consisting of separate parts. The concept of the body being whole was again lost in the West, although retained in the East in half the population of the world.

It was only in the 1960s in the West that alternative thinking in medicine, art and the environment took root again. Alternative, Holistic and Complimentary Medicine looked at the entire body as one and its functions were all interlinked. The worldwide history of medicine is covered in more detail in my "Integrated Health Bible" Chapter 2.

I belong to the group of doctors who integrated conventional and traditional medicine. My maternal grandfather was a doctor and Homoeopath so he too integrated medicine. I coined the phrase "Integrated Medicine" in 1982 as the future medical model. A doctor who has full training in conventional or Allopathic Medicine, if also specialised in Complimentary or Traditional Medical disciplines like Acupuncture, Homoeopathy, Ayurveda, Herbal Medicine, Osteopathy, Naturopathy etc, can be called an "Integrated Medical Physician". Most such doctors will prefer one angle to another so some doctors may choose to practice Acupuncture while others may choose Chiropractic or Herbal Medicine.

My model of diagnosis and treatment is as follows: for Diagnosis I use the Tongue, Pulse, Iridology, Eardology (examination of the ears) and General Examination. As a doctor I will look for tests, scans, x-rays whenever necessary. My treatment plan includes diet, massage, therapeutic yoga and other traditional therapy. But above all I treat the patient as a whole individual. My general motto is "Treat the Diseased, not the Disease".

The Hippocratic "Regimen Therapy" is the backbone of my Lifestyle Programme, which is so beautifully executed in my clinical Spa in Tuscany, Italy. Everyone has to be on a diet, have neck and marma massage, do yoga and other exercises (walk in the hills, swim in the hypersaline pool, gym exercises). The Innate Healing Power is thus aroused and sets the cure in motion. Additional therapies with supplements, natural remedies, specific massages etc complete the job.

In my London Clinic, I diagnose and recommend the Lifestyle Programme and other colleagues do the specific treatments with acupuncture, herbal medicine, psychological therapies etc

# Chapter 14 – Diet

The exact dietary plan varies from region to region as people have different eating habits and the recommendations will naturally vary.

## Basic Principles

The diet should exclude foods that cause damage to the body or interfere with digestion, if consumed in excess. Digestion takes place in an acid medium in the stomach (in the presence of stomach acid) and in an alkaline medium (created by bile from liver and pancreatic juice). If there is too much stomach acid then the digestion will slow down as the body has to wait for adequate alkali production in the form of Bile and Pancreatic juice before the food mass can be released into the small intestine. The acid is too corrosive for the lining of the intestine so it has to neutralize quickly in the small intestine.

Acid helps to break down food mass and the stomach wall can then churn and make it into a pulp (chyle) so that the rest of the digestion can take place without a hitch. If we eat too fast, then the stomach has to churn more which means that digestion will require more energy. Moreover, the stomach will need to produce more juice for making the food pulp. Those who eat very fast have problems with excess acidity in the stomach.

In the alkaline medium in the intestine, finer digestion of fats, carbohydrates and proteins takes place. Soon after digestion the intestine absorbs lipids, sugars and amino acids, which are the finest units of fats, carbohydrates and proteins, respectively. After digestion the waste has to be eliminated regularly.

# The Candida and Yeast Factors

In Nature there was always peaceful coexistence amongst bacteria, viruses and fungus, the three main invaders of our bodies. Then man discovered penicillin in the middle of the last century. It was a powerful fungal toxin synthesised commercially, to kill off all sorts of bacteria. Although it was a useful weapon against invading bacteria, doctors began to misuse it and in the 60s they used penicillin for everything from infections to allergies. As the bacteria mutated or became resistant, Medicine discovered more powerful antibiotics.

During this war between medicine and bacteria, antibiotics helped fungus and viruses to become more powerful. A fungal product (antibiotic) was used to fight bacteria and so fungi gained the upper hand. Viruses were too small and complicated so for a long time (before interferon was discovered) there was no real defence against them.

When I was a medical student in the 70s, bacterial dysentery, pneumonia, meningitis and other infections were very common. Nowadays infections like viral pneumonia, meningitis, gastric flu, glandular fever, viral hepatitis, cold sores, herpes, HIV etc are more common. Similarly, fungal infections of the nails, hair roots, mouth (ulcers), thrush, candidiasis, athlete's foot etc have also become very common. Thus, viruses and fungi as the main invaders of the body have replaced bacteria.

Brewer's yeast was a common supplement for vitamin B deficiency but today the intake of yeast causes major digestive problems. Yeast in the gut, in excess, produces toxic alcohols. Uncontrolled brewing in the gut is the main cause of gas, abdominal pain, bloating and other digestive problems. Sometimes the alcohol level in blood is quite high due to excess gut-yeast fermentation.

When you consume too much yeast you are also likely to get fungal infections as the fungi in the body have their own fraternity as they help each other. Thus you can get candida (Candida Albicans) infections in the mouth, gut, vagina, around the anus etc Candida overgrowth can cause chronic fatigue, eczema, Urticaria, dandruff, seborrhoea dermatitis (red patches on the face), some forms of Rosacea, red cheeks or noses etc The intake of sugar helps the candida and yeast overgrowth in the gut. If one takes oral antibiotics for a prolonged period, the useful gut bacteria are destroyed and opportunistic candida infections in the gut and other surfaces develop. That is why one gets thrush after a long course of antibiotics.

Thus it is potentially dangerous to consume excess fungal products, especially if you have had recurrent thrush, bloating, mouth ulcers, athlete's foot, alopecia (hair loss in patches) on the scalp, dandruff etc. I am against the intake of fungi, yeast, fungal products and excess sugar that feeds them. You must avoid or at least moderate: yeast bread (soda bread, unleavened bread are OK), pizza, pitta, nan bread, beer, yeast-spread, gravy granules (instant), cheese (hard and fungal), mushrooms, Russian kvas, malt drinks, chocolates, cakes and sweets.

Basically, the fungi yeast etc are parasites even though they taste good and add flavour to bread, soups, cheeses etc By living off the body in the gut, they do deprive you, as do worms and parasites, of some essential nutrients. Some mushrooms can kill you, blind you and some can potentially paralyse you. Edible fungi have their toxins too, except that their direct effect on the body is not noticeable. We do not know the extent to which fungi damage our body and I do not know of any study on that. For example, the yeast in the gut produces a range of toxic alcohol that goes straight to the liver. What happens next over a long period of time is anyone's guess. The extreme drowsiness that follows an hour or so after a good sandwich or carbohydrate meal is a noticeable symptom. This is due to the toxic alcohol from the gut.

If you eat mushrooms, pizza, low yeast-containing bread etc in moderation and occasionally these need not be a problem, as the body seems to cope with it. It's the regular and excessive use of fungal products that cause the problem.

There are several products you could be intolerant to in the course of your lifetime. You will know such products because you will probably get diarrhoea, bloating, gas, headaches, itchy palate or Urticaria every time you eat such a product. Avoid them as far as possible. It's not worth putting your body through such discomfort or agony just for the sake of some nice taste or pleasure.

For a European Diet Plan I use a simple scheme:

| Avoid, especially in excess | Reason |
|---|---|
| Yeast-products | Fungus |
| Cheese, mushrooms | Fungus |
| Orange, lemon, pineapple | Acid |
| White wine | Acid |
| Beer | Fungus |
| Chillies, nuts in excess | Acid |
| Preserved food | Acid /Chemicals |
| Sugar, chocolates | Feeds fungus |
| Coffee | Stimulant, often disrupts digestion |
| Foods you are intolerant to | Obviously |

Additionally, I advise the following: Eat slowly and drink water at least 45 minutes after meals so that the stomach juice is not diluted. After lunch, rest a while to allow the stomach to receive maximum energy to carry out the process of churning the food. If you have an opportunity for a siesta in the afternoon or lie down after lunch lie on your left side for 15 minutes to allow stomach juice to collect for digestion and then lie on your right, as this is where the stomach has the muscles that churn your food. After dinner, walk a bit, especially if you've had a late dinner. By walking or doing mild exercises, you stimulate the mechanical parts of the digestion, i.e. churning the food. Once you fall asleep, the body will switch off most of the digestive activities because it has to carry out repair work and rest the brain that has been active all day long. My grandfather used to say, "After lunch rest a while, after dinner walk a mile".

Many patients ask me what they should eat. My experience shows that if you avoid the foodstuffs that are bad or potentially harmful to you the digestive system will cope very well. It has a great capacity to rectify the minor damage caused by foodstuffs. It is amazing how I have helped thousands with my simple dietary plan, mentioned above. For details of Nutrition and Individual ailments refer to my Nutrition Bible. It is a book that also went on to be a bestseller in the UK and I enjoyed writing it.

To aid the process of quick healing and improving digestion I recommend my favourite Detox Tea. It is a blend of herbs that are traditionally used in India for various types of common ailments. Its ingredients are the Indian herbs Chiratha, Kadu or Kutki, Amla, Neem and Liquorice. Only half a teaspoon full of this herbal mixture is used. It is soaked in a cup of hot water at night and drunk on an empty stomach in the morning. It is bitter and no sweets are allowed afterwards. The residue is thrown away. Since it is used in such a small dose the chances of any side effects are negligible. In fact, I haven't recorded a single case where someone has had any complication. The taste may cause nausea in the beginning but one gets used to it after a couple of tries. Detox Tea helps to neutralise the excess acid in the stomach, prevents the growth of candida and yeast in the gut and helps the liver to secrete bile. It does lower the blood sugar level and occasionally people feel slightly light-headed for a few minutes. Some of my Diabetic Type II patients use it regularly and are pleased with the results. It suppresses appetite and so helps in a gentle weight loss programme. In the Castel Monastero and MITA Resort Srl, Italy Spa, Detox Tea is an extremely popular drink. People hate the taste but love the benefits.

I do recommend people to eat fruits and vegetables. If possible one should have a glass of carrot, apple, root ginger, mint leaves and celery juice. This gives one the enzymes that the digestive system so often needs and it also provides the body with fresh vitamins and micro-elements.

Pomegranate and sweet lime (found in South Asia) with a distinct sweet-sour taste and a specific bitter aftertaste, are my favourites. My grandfather, a doctor-homoeopath, often spoke about these juices as elixir of health and energy. My mother, his doting daughter, learnt a lot of his favourite recipes and remedies. She said that drinking fresh coconut water after meals aids digestion. I am sure there are fruits and berries all over the world which have a beneficial effect on digestion.

# Chapter 15 – Massage

Massage is an essential part of my Healing Technique. In the Orient, massage techniques like Shiatsu (Japanese), Tuina (Chinese), Marma (Indian), Thai etc were more therapeutic than relaxing as they are often painful. Swedish massage uses kneading and rubbing techniques and is therefore purely relaxing. Greek and Turkish massage use pummelling, slapping, rubbing and kneading techniques etc which are also therapeutic in nature.

## Benefits of massage

Muscles form the bulk of the body, a fact all too often neglected in the university Medical Anatomy year. Every movement in the body as well as standing and sitting requires the participation of the muscles and until you fall into deep sleep, the muscles are in full tone. They need ample rest to replenish their energy and rid their bulk of lactic acid, which is a by-product of excessive muscle use and poor supply of oxygen. This lactic acid can cause cramp and fatigue in muscles. Massage gets more blood into the muscles and therefore more oxygen, which instantly converts lactic acid into carbon dioxide and water.

The muscles produce maximum amounts of energy in the body. Massage is a good way of nurturing the muscles, replenishing their nutrients and keeping them toned. Exercises do similar things if they are not too strenuous (then you lose energy) and are accompanied by breathing as in Yoga and Pilates.

Massage relieves aches and pains, creating very positive sense of "feel good factor". The skin's surface is a powerful sensory organ linked to various emotions in the body. I have tried to map it and it's quite amazing how humans and animals touch each other to generate such emotions and affection. Self-touch, other than in the erogenous zones and genitalia, does not produce the same emotions. The armpit, neck, belly area, soles of feet, the area above the hips etc produce laughter (tickling sensation). The scalp induces deep relaxation and sleep. The nape of the neck and back produce "goose bumps" and sense of excitement. The areas behind the ears, lips, breasts, nipples, pubic area, the inner surface of thighs, genitalia are erogenous zones. Tickling the hair within canals of the nostrils and ears cause anger.

Therapeutic massage is used to treat Repetitive Strain Injury (as in overuse of computer, writing, physical work, sports etc), joint pain, backache, headache, stress, insomnia etc.

# The Ali Technique

Having realised that the neck holds the secret to our health, well-being and illnesses, I developed a special massage, manipulative and yoga technique to treat the neck. The idea was to improve the supply of blood and cerebral spinal fluid (brain fluid) to the brain. With some caution, one can also massage the neck on one's own. It is best, however, if someone else does the massage.

When you massage the neck from the back, there is one golden rule to follow: ***stay behind the line between the top of the shoulder and the ear*** and you will do any damage to the major arteries, nerves and the windpipe, which are located in the front of the neck.

The neck massage can be done effectively and safely along 6 lines starting from the hairline and ending on top of the shoulder. The first pair of lines originates behind the ears. Using the thumb on one side and the four fingers on the other grab the neck. Rotate the thumb and fingers and slide them down to the top of the shoulder. You might feel hard bones and some may stick out prominently. That is the sign of disalignment of the cervical vertebrae. These bony protrusions are often painful to touch. Massage them gently at first and then increase the pressure. Massage all of them downwards and upwards till they become less sore.

Then move a couple of centimetres towards the spine of the vertebrae and you will feel the tight muscles of the neck. Massage upwards or downwards along the body of the muscles. Some individual muscle bundles may be more sensitive than others. Use your thumb on one side and four fingers on the other to massage the muscles along their bulk.

Finally move towards the centre of the spine and massage the muscles that lie on either side of the axis of the spine. Some of these muscles are painful especially if the person had neck traumas or used computers a lot or had whiplash injury. These muscles help to keep the chin up and maintain posture and maintain posture and so they are often quite tender.

Using the thumb, massage horizontally along the hair line where the tendons of the neck muscles are attached to the occiput (skull bone). They are very sore to touch especially if the neck muscles are tight. These tendons are the extensions of muscles so they often tear and get strained with neck injuries. Massage all these tendons, till the pain eases.

Massage the areas below the ear and behind the angle of the lower jaw (mandible). This is the area where the vertebral arteries come out of the cervical or neck canals and enters the brain. This area is covered with a thick sheath of membrane that protects these vital arteries. Massage with the thumb but use gentle pressure. This helps to instantly improve a headache if one has one.

Massage the jaw and the temples, which helps to improve circulation of the Cerebro Spinal Fluid that bathes the brain surface, supplying it with glucose and some dissolved oxygen.

I recommend using my Joint Oil or Back Massage oil which is a blend containing Mustard Oil, Clove Oil, Sesame Oil, Winter Green etc You can prepare some at home using organic sesame oil (50 ml), clove oil (5 ml), mustard oil (30 ml), black cumin seed oil (Kolonji, 15 ml). The other oils used in my formula are Ayurvedic.

Take half a teaspoonful of the oil and rub it between the palms till it becomes warm. This activates the ingredients and helps it to penetrate the skin to reach the muscles. The clove oil eliminates pain while the others help to relieve inflammation of the muscles.

You must remember that these muscles help to hold your head up vertically to maintain the posture. The bones of the vertebrae, skull, and shoulder just provide the surfaces to which the muscles are attached. When you fall asleep in a car or train, your head drops in all sorts of directions as the muscles lose power. The cervical spine cannot hold your head up on its own. The head is the single heaviest organ in the body followed by the liver. It rests on a pair of pivotal joints on the top of the first vertebra of the neck. Almost 2/3 of the head lies in front of these joints and 1/3 behind, thus it is front heavy. The front part has the bulk of the brain, facial bones, eyes, tongue, teeth etc So, like in a seesaw, the front part of the head would naturally tilt forward, but thanks to the neck muscles as the back and the chin is kept up. If we are up and about for 16 hours a day, the neck muscles work continuously during that period. By the end of the day they become stiff and quite sore from the lactic acid. Unless we massage them (passive) or exercise them (active), they would add to the problems of the neck. The joints would be stiffer and the discs would degenerate, shrinking the length of the neck, which can reduce blood flow to the brain and cause trouble.

Massaging the shoulder and upper back are also very important. The Trapezius muscle of the upper back helps to support the head and keeps the chin up. Thus the shoulder and upper back should also be included in the massage technique performed by a partner or therapist. If possible, the therapist should use a towel to grip the occiput (back of the skull) and pull the head away from the body with a mild traction. One should breathe deeply while this procedure is carried out for a minute or so.

I have my own manipulation technique which can only be taught to medically qualified practitioners or osteopaths and chiropractors. I do not do vigorous manipulations of the neck or adjustments of the misaligned vertebrae. Some therapists do just that and do not prepare the muscles of the neck and shoulder. In some cases they will have several patients lying on the couches and spend a few minutes adjusting the neck vertebrae. Patients feel good instantly but have to return to the therapist, again and again as they need repeated adjustments which is an expensive experience.

The joints of the vertebrae dislocate or are misaligned or subluxated because of the muscles which create torsion and "pull" the joints "out". Take the example of the whiplash, the movement of the neck, first forward and then backward, dislocates the joints. The muscles in the cervical spine also get injured as a result of this. The therapist should work on such tight muscles and then gently adjust the joints. The results are more long term and beneficial to the patient.

Some people habitually "click" their own neck and adjust their neck several times a day to "feel good". The joints dislocate within a few hours, and need readjustment. In my opinion, the more you manipulate the neck the more there is a need to do this.

Ask your osteopath or chiropractor to massage the various muscles of the neck and back. Tell them also to work on the ligaments of the facet joints. After that they can manipulate the joints. They may not like to be told what to do, but you must be polite.

# Chapter 16 – Therapeutic Yoga

The West interpreted yoga as a series of exercises … but the fact is that yoga is a suitable form of safe exercises and relaxation for every one of all ages.

Although yoga is relatively new to the West, it has a long and venerable tradition in the East. It dates back to at least 3000 BC and has been practised in India to promote physical and spiritual health.

Yoga was popularised in the West during the 1960s by a number of gurus, spiritual leaders and philosophers who promoted all things Indian. Their approach to life appealed hugely to many rock stars, like The Beatles, Rolling Stones and to many celebrities because it contrasted starkly with the materialistic approach to life which predominated in the West at the time.

The West interpreted yoga as a series of exercises and thought of it in much the same way as other forms of physical workout. What's more, many people worried it would take years to master the many complicated positions. The fact is that yoga is a suitable form of safe exercises and relaxation for every one of all ages.

Over the last few decades' yogic exercise has become increasingly popular. Thanks to the efforts of some celebrities, and the modern preoccupation with fitness and stress management. Yet, in its original form, yoga is so much more than just a system of exercise and for those in the know, yoga is a whole way of life, encompassing diet, massage, relaxation and meditation.

It regulates your breathing, increases your energy, helps to overcome fatigue, relieves aches and pains in the joints, improves your posture, the circulation of blood and lymph and calms the mind. As well as being a great way to stay in shape, it also promotes the body's natural healing powers, and so it can be used to treat a wide range of health problems, both physical and emotional – hence the description "therapeutic".

We can survive for a while without food or water, but not without air as we need oxygen to metabolise the food we eat and to create energy. This is generally an involuntary process, meaning that most of the time you are not aware that you are doing it but yoga teaches you to breathe voluntarily.

# Yogic (Hatha) Breathing

When you breathe normally, only about two thirds of the air in your lungs are exchanged. The other third remains stagnant in your respiratory system because the lungs and the bronchial tract do not collapse totally during exhalation. When you practice yogic breathing, however, you can replace more of the air in your lungs. Yogic breathing is deeper and more efficient, therefore more beneficial to the body.

Yoga teaches you to breathe slowly and deeply, helping you to deal with stress. The more anxious, you are, the more erratic your breathing becomes. If you voluntarily slow your breathing into a deep rhythmic pattern, prolonging the time between inhalation and exhalation, oxygen absorption becomes more efficient. The blood returning to the heart from the lungs is therefore more enriched with oxygen, which triggers the brain to slow the heart rate. This can really help you to calm down. It also helps to keep your brain cells healthy and active, which is particularly important as you grow older -- your brain tissues need three times more oxygen than the rest of your body. The two exercises, which I therefore recommend to start any yoga session, are Cleansing Breath and Alternate Nostril Breathing.

**Cleansing Breath**, (should not be attempted if you have high blood pressure, a hernia or ulcer or prolapsed organs in the lower abdomen).

1.  Stand or sit comfortably with your arms relaxed by your sides. Straighten your upper back and pull your shoulders back. Close your mouth and look straight ahead.

2.  Breathe out forcefully, pulling your stomach in. Repeat 25 times.

# Alternate Nostril Breathing

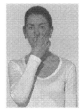

1. Place your thumb on your right nostril to close it and breathe in deeply through your left nostril.

2. Then close your left nostril with your middle finger and release your thumb. Breathe out, completely through your right nostril. Feel your chest muscles relaxing and your shoulders dropping away from your neck as you exhale.

Then breathe in through your right nostril.

3. Close your right nostril with the thumb, release your finger and breathe out through the left nostril. You have now completed one cycle.

4. Continue for 3 to 5 minutes. Then relax for a few minutes.

# Yoga Involving the Neck

Many yoga exercises impinge upon the neck, while not being designed specifically for it.

## Prone Exercises

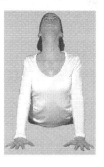

### Lie on your stomach

#### Cobra-full

1. Place your palms flat on the floor beside your shoulders.

2. Take a deep breath in, lift your torso up and look up to the ceiling. The entire body is arched back with the help of the back muscles and the arms give it minimal support.

3. Breathe out, and gently return to the original position with forehead on the floor. Repeat this five times.

## Cobra-half

Put your elbows by your sides. Take a deep breath in and raise your head, looking up. Hold your breath for five seconds, and slowly come down, breathing out. The forehead should touch the floor. Repeats this five times.

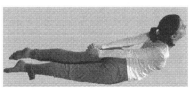

## Swing

1. Lie on your front, clasp your hands, put them behind you.

2. Take a deep breath in and raise your torso as well as your legs up in the air. Hold your breath in this position.

3. Arch your back, to look up and stretch your toes out. You should feel tightness along the back muscles, the seat muscles and the hamstrings and calves. Hold this position for a count of five.

4. Return to the normal position, breathing out again and placing your forehead on the floor. Repeat five times.

## Lie on your back

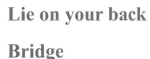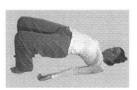

## Bridge

1. Lie on your back, bend your knees.

2. Take a deep breath in and raise your pelvic as high as you can.

3. Draw the chin closer to your chest. Hold breath for five counts.

4. Put your hips down and breathe out.

5. Repeat this five times.

## Spinal Twist

1. Extend arms at shoulder level.

2. Bring knees up with feet on the floor.

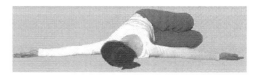

3. Take a deep breath and turn your head to the left (ear should touch floor), while lowering your knees to the floor on the right (opposite direction).

4. Breathe out, and then breathe in and out very gently. As you do this you must make sure that your shoulders are flat on the floor. You should feel the twist in your spine and your knees will gradually descend to the floor as muscular tension is released from the lower back.

5. Repeat the exercise turning your head to the right and letting your knees come down to the floor on the left.

6. Repeat two or three times on each side.

This exercise will twist the spine to release spasm of muscles as well as help to align facet joints of vertebrae which get dislocated. This is a self-manipulative technique.

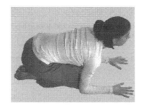

## Midway exercises

### Turtle-pose

1. Kneel and sit back on your heels. Place both elbows by the sides of the knees by bending forwards. Put your forehead on the floor.

2. Take a deep breath in and raise your head and look as far up as you can, keeping the elbows on the floor. Put your chest forwards. Hold your breath in this position for five seconds.

3.   Slowly breathe out and return to the original position.

4.   Repeat this five times.

## Standing exercises

### Arching back

1.   Stand with feet together. Tighten your seat muscles. Breathe in.

2.   Place both hands on the buttocks and push it forward. As you do  this, look up, arching your back. Do not bend your knees while doing this.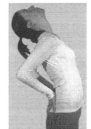

3.   Hold your breath for five seconds and return to the original position on breathing out.

4.   Repeat this five times. You should be able to feel the tension in your lower back, and the release of it when you return to the original position.

### Arms arch

1.   Stand with your feet together. Take a deep breath in and hold your breath.

2.   Entwine your fingers behind your back, tighten your seat muscles and pull both arms down as if to touch your heels. Arch your back as you do this and look up. You should get the feeling that your back muscles and the muscles of your arms are taut.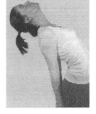

3.   Hold this position for a count of five. Breathe out and return to the normal position.

# Yoga Specifically for the Neck

## Neck Twist

1. Look ahead and grip your right shoulder (in the middle, not at the extremity) with the left hand. Place the right arm behind your back.
2. Take a deep breath in and rotate your head towards the right, while simultaneously pulling the right shoulder forward with the left hand. Hold your breath for five seconds. By doing this you will feel the stretch in the muscles of the right side of your neck and a release of tension in its joints.
3. Return to the original position.
4. Repeat the same with the other side.
5. Do this five times in each direction.

This exercise will strengthen the muscles of the neck; improve movement of the neck in both directions, releasing the stiffness and shifting vertebrae that are out of alignment back into their original positions. This often acts like self-manipulation.

## Head roll

1. Bend your head so that the chin touches your chest.

2. Rotate the head in a clockwise direction, making sure parts of your head (chin, lower jaw, back of the head) touch your chest and the chances of dizziness are minimized.

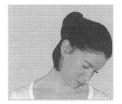

3. Do this five times, and repeat in the anticlockwise direction.

This exercise will help to grind osteophytes or calcium deposits that so often settle on the joint services all around. This releases the joints from stiffness.

Whether it says so or not, breathing should be co-ordinated with each movement in all the exercises.

After your exercises, lie down and relax for five minutes. Deep relaxation is described fully in my Ultimate Back Book page 114, but basically it amounts to lying on your back in a quiet place with eyes closed; breathing deeply; concentrating on something abstract; being aware of your muscles becoming warm and relaxing all over your body; imagine your heart is slowing down. When ready take more deep breaths, open your eyes and rise slowly, avoiding anything stressful for as long as you can.

# Chapter 17 – Where to go for treatment of the neck

The Ali Technique is one of the best tools for treating the neck and restoring all its functions. The neck holds the head, helps it turn in different directions, protects the most vital blood vessels and nerves, facilitates the nourishment and protection of the brain by regulating the circulation of brain fluid (CSF) and maintains the crucial link between the brain and the rest of the body. The neck is the most vital structure of the body and its functions have to be continually supported.

The Ali Technique is in practice, a family art of treatment. My brothers, some nephews and cousins, distant relatives, a few members of my village near Calcutta, some doctors who trained under me, some staff at The Castel Monastero in Tuscany, Italy and Forte Village in Sardinia, Italy and my sons know the technique. Previous staff therapists of my Integrated Medical Centres in London and New Delhi, and my Sagoor Charity Clinic in The Kangra Valley in the Himalayas follow my technique. My family members, however, know the finer aspects of my technique as they have lot of experience and have worked closely with me. What pleases me most is that The Ali Technique as a family art will survive and continue to bring relief to the thousands. Hopefully, a training school will help to teach therapists this art.

The massage technique described in the previous chapter demonstrated in various DVDs, in my eBook and explained in my other books is adequate for relief of many symptoms of the Ali Syndrome and maintenance of the functions of the neck.

Here are other methods that help in the treatment of some of the symptoms of The Ali Syndrome and in preventing them:

1.  Sports Massage. Qualified therapists who treat sports injury with massage.

2.  Deep Tissue Massage.

3.  Shiatsu of the neck and shoulder areas.

4.  Osteopaths and Chiropractors who use massage first and  manipulation later.

5.  Thai Massage.

6.  Ayurvedic, Head and Neck Massage.

7.  Traction of the neck with low weights and controlled intermittent traction (used very rarely now).

8.  Highly qualified Acupuncturists who are able to relieve neck Traction

All the above Practitioners and Therapists should be properly qualified and have minimum five years experience in a clinic and not in a spa (unless trained).

Please check my website for the list of Therapists who are directly or indirectly trained by me or my family members.

www.drmali.com

Shortly after the release of this book, training courses will be offered to doctors, osteopath, physiotherapist, qualified massage and sports injury therapist.

Hopefully, there will be more therapists.

Here are the contact details of our centres:

**Integrated Medical Centre, UK**
121, Crawford Street, London, W1U 6BE, UK
e: info@integratedmed.co.uk
http://www.integratedmed.co.uk/

**Integrated Medical Centre, India**
D-40, East of Kailash, New Delhi – 110065, India
t: +91-11-4652 2945
e: imc-delhi@msn.com

**Castel Monastero, Italy**
Near Siena, Tuscany, Italy
http://www.castelmonastero.com/

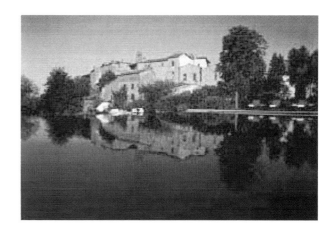

**Forte Village Resort**
Sardinia – Italy
http://www.fortevillageresort.com/

**For training courses contact:**
e: info@theneckconnection.com

# Chapter 18 – The Other Neck Connection

The neck is located below the cranium or skull, which houses the headquarters of the nervous system - the computer centre.

From the space below each of the seven cervical vertebrae, a pair of nerves emerges from the spinal cord and goes to various parts of the head, shoulder, arm, hand, and figure.

Thus compression of nerve roots emerging from the spinal cord at the neck level can cause pain, burning, tingling, electric currents and numbness in the corresponding part of the upper body. Usually if the nerve is severely pressed for a long time, they begin to lose their conductivity; the result is numbness (loss of feeling). The other symptoms like tingling, burning etc are due to active irritation or compression.

The cervical vertebrae have disks to cushion them. These are located between the bodies of the vertebrae. If there is any whiplash, trauma or continuous wear and tear, these discs bulge and can scratch or irritate nerve roots, causing the above symptoms.

If one suffers from osteoporosis, the initial bone loss starts at the level of the neck, which is the most "used" part of the spine and the degeneration of the discs cause the neck to shrink so the person loses height. It's only later that bone loss may appear in the hip and lower spine. When the neck, shrinks, there is often a lot of nerve irritation at random causing all sorts of nerve pains, tingling, burning, numbness etc in the neck, shoulder, arms, hands and fingers. The vertebral arteries are also compressed and, as a result, the patient suffers from extreme fatigue, dizziness, imbalance, tinnitus, anxiety, memory loss etc

Sometimes the degenerated discs bulge into the spinal canal, rather than protrude out. This causes stenosis or narrowing of the spinal canal. Occasionally the bulge may touch or damage the spinal cord causing serious neurological problems.

## Weakness in the leg caused by damage in the spinal cord in the neck region

A lady in her 70s came to see me with some strange sensations in her leg and she often lost power in her left foot while walking and tripped. Sometimes she had to take extra care while climbing stairs as, for no apparent reason, her foot would drop and she would trip. I examined her and found no apparent cause of any back problem but I suspected that something was wrong with her neck as she had frequent headaches and dizziness. I sent her for an MRI scan of the neck and result showed that a bony growth was touching and indenting the spinal cord. I recommended she go for neurosurgery. This cured her problem.

## Sylvester Stallone and the neck connection

Sylvester Stallone, the famous Hollywood Star who is one of the top action heroes, took numerous direct hits on the face and head while filming the Rocky and Rambo films. He had sustained heavy injuries to the neck and shoulder areas and the pain was so excruciating that he had to wear a neck brace to sleep at night. He was on the strongest painkillers you could find and surgeons wanted to operate immediately. He invited me to Los Angeles and I started working on his neck muscles, facet joints, tendons and ligaments twice a day. The pain was severe but he let me treat him. After 6 days the pain was gone and he was greatly relieved. Being an exercise-conscious person he did regular exercises and controlled the symptoms.

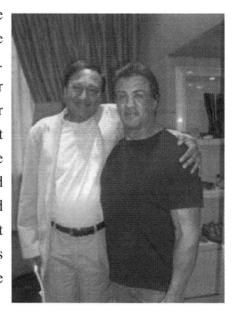

### Shahrukh Khan

Shahrukh Khan, known as the King of Bollywood, is an incredible man of courage, tolerance and great intelligence. As an actor he did many of the stunts himself and therefore had to endure several injuries. In one film, for a more dramatic effect, he kicked the ground to scoop some dirt on to the face of a wicked villain. Little did he know that there was a stone in the ground and so he smashed his big toe but gave a perfect shot. He is a great dancer

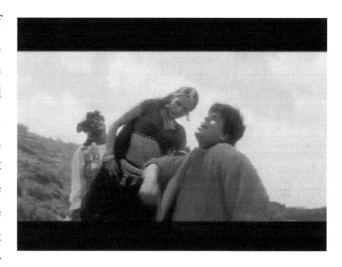

and years of repetitive injuries gave him gave him some knee problems. He continues to do action scenes like jumping from a tall building, moving between two trains running at full speed while being suspended from a crane, doing somersaults, doing fight scenes with the body strapped to wires for special effect etc.

His neck injuries were top of the list. In one movie 'Dil Se' he danced on top of a moving train and while filming this song he had to move his neck sideways several thousands of time in a Sufi ritual, like those performed by Whirling Dervishes. In another film 'Devdas' where the death scene was meant to be dramatic so he lay dead on the grass as his body was discovered in the early hours of the morning. To get the perfect morning light, the director shot this important scene for 11 days, filming only a few minutes a time. A fly was shown settling on his face, as he lay motionless. That scene put a lot of strain on his neck muscles, as he had to tighten them and remain motionless, without breathing.

In another movie, he ran across the airport check-in area to stop his wife from boarding a plane as they had parted company the previous night. He jumped over a train of trolleys and landed on his back causing severe injury to the neck as there was no mattress or cushion on the other side.

I was treating him for his neck and gave him much relief in the initial phase. The later injuries made the discs in the neck pinch the nerves and he had excruciating pain going down his left arm. Finally Mr. Crockard his Neuro-Surgeon operated on him at The Wellington Hospital in London. The pain, however, continued so on the 2nd day after the surgery, Mr. Crockard gave me permission to treat him to alleviate the pain with my technique. I treated him for a month while his nerve roots healed. He played monopoly game with his friends which distracted him from the pain. After the surgery he also experienced dizziness and imbalance and these symptoms too disappeared within that period.

## Excruciating pain in the neck, shoulder and down the arm

An internationally known President of a luxury goods company was dining with the late Princess Diana and my friend, David Tang, who is well-connected in Hong Kong and London. This gentleman complained of excruciating pain in his neck, shoulder and arm and so he was going in for surgery. Both David and The Princess strongly recommended that I saw him before he had surgery. I was in the palace of an Arab Head of State and had mistakenly forgotten to switch off the phone. David ordered me to return to London "immediately" (He is always funny and very witty). I explained where I was and so he told me to see his friend ASAP.

I saw the gentleman after a few days but he was very sceptical, as he had already seen top specialists who suggested surgery. After the very first session he had some relief so he gave me the benefit of the doubt and invited me to his summer house.

I put him on a diet and treated him with my technique. The pain disappeared after a week and he came of all drugs as he could sleep comfortably. Since then he became one of my greatest advocates and through him I saw dozens of very important people all over the world. I am deeply indebted to him for appreciating my technique and skill. Sometimes you need angels like him to get you to where you are. So many people were saved from back and other operations because of his recommendation.

Like all joints, the facet joints of the cervical spine are subject to arthritis. Most frequently it is due to wear and tear or old age and sometimes, it is due to rheumatoid arthritis when the joints become very stiff and painful especially in the morning.

Sometimes the neck can go into spasm, on one side. You then get a "crooked neck" and this condition is called Torticollis. It often happens due to sleeping awkwardly at night and you wake up in the morning with a crooked neck. Neck massages and poultices with hot salt are good treatments for Torticollis.

## Stretched nerves of the neck

A famous Oscar-award winning Hollywood actor had a car accident in which he injured the nerves of the neck. As a result there was paralysis in the left arm and with excellent physiotherapy his arm began to move but his hands remained out of actions. I met him at a party in Abu Dhabi almost 3 years after the accident. When he told me about the accident, the excruciating pain he had in his arm and the loss of movement in his hand. I began to treat him in full glaze of hundreds of celebrities at that party. That night he slept very well, without much pain so I saw him again for 2 hrs. The following day and explained what I did. He said "I trust you". I went to Los Angeles a few times and treated his neck and arm. The wrist and fingers began to move and the horrible pain that used to keep him awake at night reduced considerably. I treat him every couple of months for a few days and he is making a steady progress. The good news is that he continues to act in movies.

# Chapter 19 – Spontaneous Healing with The Ali Technique

## If the Hypothalamus-Pituitary region controls all autonomous functions in the body, then it must also control healing.

Improved blood supply to the subconscious brain and patients' participation in their own healthcare improves general healing. Again, by using logic, we can see how that works. If the Hypothalamus-Pituitary region controls all autonomous functions in the body, then it must also control healing. The general well-being, increased energy, better sleep etc with diet, massage, yoga and supplements helps the body to heal better.

### Fracture in Tibia bone that didn't heal for 6 months

An English woman in her late forties came to see me with a fracture in her tibia bone of the right leg. She had a compound fracture with many splinter bones. For almost 6 months and so she could not walk properly because of pain so she put on weight as well. I changed her die and asked her to drink marrow bone soup (marrow bone boiled in slow heat for 2 hours to get the calcium and gelatine out), eat fresh fruits and green salad. I gave her weekly treatment of the neck and the thigh and calf muscles (avoiding the fractured area). After 8 weeks she went to have an x-ray. The doctors were very pleased in the hospital as they saw evidence of new bone tissue and after 8 more weeks the bone healed completely. The general well being accelerated her healing.

When Wayne Rooney, the English football star, who plays for Manchester United Team, had a fracture of the metatarsal bone in his foot, the whole nation was in despair as it was just before the 2006 World Cup. I suggested my treatment through a Press release, covered only by The Sun newspaper. Then I was called by Sky News TV to give my suggestion. They interviewed me for 5 minutes to explain what I could do to make him heal quickly. Hundreds of patients with fractures of various types contacted me after the TV interview. I gave them my entire treatment plan: neck massage, diet and self-massage of the area above and below the fracture to improve local circulation. Many reported positive results within a short period of time.

## Infected left Humerus bone

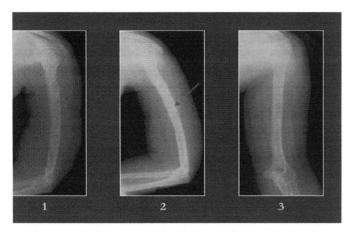

X-rays of the arm of the lady with bone infection

An Indian lady could not get a Visa to join her husband in Canada as she failed the crucial medical test of the Canadian High Commission in Delhi because of an infected left Humerus bone (arm). The infection (Osteomyelitis) produced pus that oozed out from that arm so she used to dress the wound and was permanently on antibiotic. The lady came to see me in desperation from Punjab, some 8 hours journey from Delhi. I suggested a diet of juices, cottage cheese, soaked almonds and some protein powder, as she was a strict vegetarian. I taught her relative how to do the neck and the arm massage. She followed my programme religiously as she had faith in me.

After 6 months she came to visit me in my Delhi clinic and showed me a piece of bone in a jar. She also gave me some x-rays of her arm which showed the process of healing in sequence. Her body rejected a piece of infected bone and you could see the healing in progress. I still have those x-rays which I have used in my public lectures. She now lives in Canada with her husband. This was a true example of how the body heals itself, provided the innate healing power is nurtured. Her x-rays are shown below.

## Brain Tumour (Glioma)

A cloth merchant from Delhi requested me to see his ailing father who had brain tumour (Glioma). I flew to Amritsar in Northern India from Delhi and went to see the patient. When I saw him, he was having one of the frequent seizures. His face was swollen and he had lost a lot of weight and he had constant nausea, sickness and headaches. It was obvious he was dying and there was nothing I could do. Since I had gone there I thought I should at least try to make him feel better. Sometimes you treat serious patients on compassionate grounds.

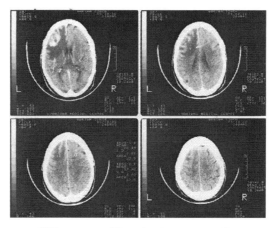

CT scans of brain tumor patient

I suggested, Khichdi rice (rice cooked with lentils, till it becomes like porridge or kedgeree), carrot and apple juices and yoghurt. He was vegetarian so I couldn't even suggest eggs as a source of protein. I demonstrated the neck and shoulder massage to a relative and suggested they did the massage three times a day. I also suggested some liquid multivitamins with minerals.

After just 2 weeks, the son came to see me in my Delhi clinic. He had visited his father over the weekend and was thrilled that he had responded positively to the treatment. His seizures stopped and he could eat normal food without being sick. When you are young and have less experience, every success story makes you feel proud.

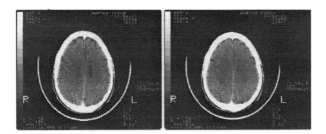

**Later CT Scans of brain tumor patient**

A few months later, he was brought to Delhi to see me. I compared his CT scan with the first one and there was a definite reduction in the tumour size and so I told them to continue the same plan of treatment: neck massage, diet, and supplements.

After a few months, he came to see me again. He was perfectly normal and looked healthy. I took him to The Aggarwal X-ray and Scan Centre in central Delhi. After the CT scan was done, Dr Sudershan Aggarwal, who knew me well asked me how I treated him. He was very surprised, as the Tumour had completely disappeared and he added that he had never seen anything like that in his entire career. He was an excellent radiologist except his technician got the left and right side mixed-up and marked the scans wrongly. In those days CT scan was in the early stage of development in India.

## Down syndrome

A little boy of one and half years with Down syndrome was brought to see me by her mother in the London clinic. She wanted to try any treatment I would suggest, as there is no other hope. Thrice a week he came to the clinic for neck massage and Marma therapy. After 6 months, he started to speak a few words and he became very alert, his concentration was good, and he developed noticeable communication skills, hardly suffered from colds and cough and became a very cheerful boy. It is his 3rd year of treatment in my London clinic and he has almost caught up with his milestones development. He has a genetic problem linked to a chromosome defect and yet he had noticeable improvement in his physical and emotional state. He didn't have any birth injury or neck trauma. There is no neck connection here as far as the cause is concerned but The Ali Technique helped his general well being.

# Multiple Sclerosis

This is a debilitating neurological disorder caused by scar tissue in the brain causing loss of coordination, difficulty in walking, tingling, numbness, spasticity, visionary problems, etc.

Several cases of Multiple Sclerosis are under our treatment. The neck treatment and Marma massage have helped them to go into remission.

## Multiple Sclerosis in remission

One young Indian lady with confirmed MS is under our treatment in London for many years. She now lives in India where the summer heat often aggravates the symptoms of muscle weakness, coordination fatigue etc. She gets occasional tingling or pain in the legs due to normal backache or sciatica, but with treatment that gets resolved. It is almost 10 years now and she has come off steroids and is in long-term remission. She hasn't had a scan to see if the plaques or "white spots" are still there in the brain. She is nervous and doesn't want to know.

## Multiple Sclerosis in remission

A lady in her forties in Rome could not walk due to lack of coordination and imbalance because of MS. The Ali Technique has stabilized her symptoms and she is able to walk, travel and work in her bikini business. She has regular treatment from me and another therapist in Rome.

# Adjuvant Cancer Therapy

About 10 years ago, when I used to write a column for *The Mail* on Sunday's coloured supplement, *YOU* magazine, a patient asked me for advice on cancer therapy. In the column I wrote about diet, juices, neck massage, meditation and some supplements as adjuvant therapy to normal medical treatment with Radio and Chemotherapy.

After a few weeks an official from The Westminster Council's Health Department in London came to see me. He served me a notice to say that I have broken the 1930 Law on promoting alternative cancer therapy, which was not officially accepted. I said that because I moved into the UK in 1991, I was not aware of any law that restricted me to publicly express my views on a health matter. I also argued that I did not recommend any chemical medicine or herbs for cancer and nor I did I claim to have a cure for cancer. He let me off after I wrote a letter of apology for writing about cancer.

As a well know practitioner of Integrated Medicine, a lot of cancer patients come to me for advice. I tell them to go through the normal medical plan of therapy with surgery when possible, chemotherapy and radiotherapy as all three have a great role to play in controlling the cancer. I suggest a therapy to counteract the side effects of such drugs, focus on well-being and 'feel-good' factor. My belief is that if we counteract the effect of chemo or radio therapy, the chances are that the body will be able to spring back to health. A strict diet (organic food where possible), vegetable and fruit juices for additional vitamins, minerals and enzymes, massage of the whole body particularly the neck and shoulder areas, yoga and meditation or relaxation, some supplements and herbal remedies; (for Candida, energy, digestive disturbances, liver functions etc) help the body and the mind. The neck massage improves sleep, eliminates symptoms of nausea, fatigue, headaches, insomnia etc (after chemotherapy) and gives a boost to the energy and the immune system. This way the patients can tolerate these strong therapies better. My programme continues even after these therapies are stopped and so we can see true remission. The patients, by participating in their own healthcare build the will to live and are not afraid of dying.

## Breast cancer in remission with integrated medical therapy

A lady with breast cancer was given 2-3 months to live as the chemotherapy didn't work and the side effects were horrendous (sickness, fainting, anxiety). It is her 4th year now and she goes through regular check-up without any sign of cancer anywhere. She went to my

Himalayan Sagoor Clinic, had 6 weeks of integrated medical therapy and continues to follow the programme.

I must warn that my treatment helps patients to cope with the conventional therapies and with the comfortable recuperation. After that the immune system takes over and patients can go into remission.

## Patient with HIV positive and Kaposi's Sarcoma

A young lady who after being infected by a boyfriend with HIV positive came to see me with Kaposi's sarcoma on her lips, which is a tumour and is caused by the Herpes virus. The tumour was removed by surgery. I suggested a therapy of diet, neck massage and supplements which she followed for 6 months. Actually, she went on to study Ayurvedic Medicine to understand her condition better. It's more than 10 years and she has not had any active leisons since then. She is HIV positive but she did not develop AIDS.

## Stress in life

A woman in her early fifties had a lot of stress in her life. A messy divorce, loss of a powerful job, financial problems, loneliness etc, ruined her life. She had total Alopecia and lost all her hair and eyebrows. She wore a head-scarf, pencilled her eyebrows and she was severely depressed. She saw several specialists and took steroids but nothing helped her condition.

Someone spoke to her about me to her so she came to see me. I was really touched by her story. I gave her a lot of encouragement and told her to change her diet, have regular neck treatments and do yoga. She was so impressed that she followed my instructions very carefully. After a few weeks, the hair started to appear on her scalp. This encouraged her to follow the programme even more religiously.

She went on my Himalayan trip and stayed on for a few more weeks. She was Indian but lived abroad all her life. With great enthusiasm she studied the culture, local tradition and their lives.

It was the best period of her life. She was carefree and studied her roots with great enthusiasm.

Whenever her grand daughter has any problems like, cradle cap that doesn't heal, colic, constipation, flu etc, she comes to see me. This baby was born with forceps and has had some problems. She has neck and body massage from her grandmother and is growing up to be a delightful and healthy child.

## Conclusion

These are individual cases but even one case is symbolic. It goes to prove that the integrated treatment has some very positive effect on the body. I will continue to accept difficult cases where medicine fails because deep in my heart I believe that I have discovered a Panacea of health. Any help I can offer to such chronic patients who are in agony is a bonus. I am doing my job as a doctor, the best I can. I believe in the Hippocratic preaching, "Physicians do not harm". My treatment has not harmed anybody, even if it has not always helped some. I strongly believe that the body can heal itself provided the conditions are laid down for it to do so.

# My Own Experience

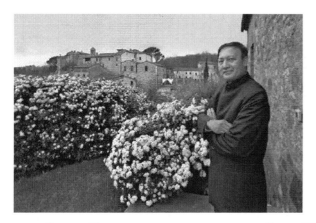

*So why did I write this book? I have had the compelling desire to reveal the importance of truly understanding and caring for the body, especially the neck ... I want to pass on what I have learned through my own experiences of neck injuries - hence this book. ...*

So why did I wrote this book? I have had the compelling desire to reveal the importance of truly understanding and caring for the body, especially neck since I was a young student in boarding school. I studied hard and suffered severe insomnia, hyperactivity and headaches. It was a Christian Brother who became concerned for my welfare and showed me the way. Now I want to pass on what I have learned through my own experiences of neck injuries - hence this book.

It all started with my maternal grandfather, who was both a doctor and a homeopath. He was a great believer in natural birth and non-invasive methods of treatment. In fact he was a true integrated medical doctor. He preferred to use homeopathic remedies rather than allopathic medicines.

I was the first born in the family and my grandfather insisted that my mother had the best midwife in the area. I was delivered in the family home near Calcutta. My mother told me, as I was the first-born, the labour was long and difficult. I realized later that my head must have been stuck in the birth canal. The contractions must have squashed my neck periodically over several hours. That is not an uncommon occurrence.

In theory I should have had some birth injuries to the neck, which would have led to a weak immune system, eczema, lack of concentration etc. However my grandfather did what was the tradition in India. For forty days both my mother and I received care from the midwife, who are called 'Dais' in India.

In the holy city of Benares on the Ganges, said to be the oldest city in India, there was a school that trained these Dais. They were taught to care for both the mother and the new born and made sure every thing was hygienic and the newborn was fed on time, bathed, sunbathed, dressed and handled carefully. The mother was also taught childcare and she allowed the necessary time to recuperate fully. She learned how to eat a good diet and to take enough rest to produce the best quality milk for the newborn.

The massage of the neck and spine rectified all the trauma and damage the newborn may have endured at birth. At the end of the 40-day period, the baby was able to hold the head up with more strength. Massage plays an important role in restoring good blood flow to the fast developing brain and result is that the child feels well, does not suffer from colds or coughs, develops at the right rate and is generally happy and alert.

My mother told me I was brought up according to my grandfather's instructions, breastfed and given the daily massage for the first year. She said I had never suffered from colic, diarrohea, infection, rash, bloating or any of the trials that new babies are so often heir to. I crawled and walked early and was a quick learner.

Could it be that my memory developed well because of that massage of the neck and shoulder area? For example, on my first birthday my grandfather gave me few present, I later learned those were gold chain and a gold waistband studded with semiprecious stones. There was a large gathering of family members and friends in his mansion to celebrate my first birthday. I remember being aware of a lot of commotion when one of the guests stole the precious gifts. It left a clear impression on me. The theft was never solved and it was a very unpleasant incident as many guests left without attending the family feast. Years later I asked my mother about the commotion and she told me the real story. She was surprised that how could I remember that incident when I was just one year old..

I can remember another incident that happened when I was about eighteen months old. I was sitting in a truck surrounded by many people shouting, "Vote for Ali". My father, a politician, in those days stood for West Bengal elections and I was taken by someone on the campaign trip. My father won the election and I remember that we had many visitors to the house. One was Dr B. C. Roy, the first chief minister of West Bengal who later became my ideal. He used to diagnose patients by looking at telltale signs on the body, tongue, pulse and eyes. Today part of my own diagnosis follows that technique.

I was a good student and was always first in my class at school. The son of a wealthy businessman died of leukaemia in my school so the father set up a scholarship in his memory for the student who achieved the best percentage of marks every year. I was the first recipient of that scholarship.

When I looked at early photographs of myself, I observed that my left eye was smaller than the right which was an indication that I had sustained some significant birth injuries and yet I didn't have any of the complications that I have mentioned in this book. The early treatment was my saviour. Sometimes when I am tired, I do find my left eye slightly shut and the asymmetry of the eyes is noticeable.

When I was eight years old I was sent to boarding school, which had been a Military Hospital during the First World War. The school was run by Christian Brothers who were strict but caring. I was there for eight years and during that time had suffered two distinct injuries. Once when I was playing grass hockey, the ball hit me hard on the nose and it bled profusely. I was dizzy afterwards for several days. When I was in class 10 I had decided that I wanted to box. I joined a group who used to go for a jog at 5.30 am every day, followed by exercises and for breakfast we had a meal of soaked horse gram (pulses), a rich source of protein used by wrestlers and sportsmen in Asia. I also ate raw egg for stamina. I was tall, skinny and had long arms for my weight and so I thought I had all the advantages to be a good boxer. The very first time I was in the ring I was punched by my opponent in the nose. I had flashes of light in my eyes, and almost lost balance and the fight was stopped. I could not smell very well for days after that incident. That was typical of the Neck Connection.

I was still young and very active so the symptoms disappeared quite quickly. It was a year later that I started getting insomnia. I would wake up at 3 am sharp and would not be able to sleep until 5 am or so and this happened on most nights. Initially I would try to divert my mind, counted sheep, imagined that I was flying like a bird over valleys and fields. Sometimes these helped but generally the routine remained the same.

Being a conscientious student I would go down at night to the study hall to read lessons. The schoolmasters were confident I would achieve a rank in the final school leaving board examination conducted by the University of Cambridge in UK. Our principal, Brother Whiting, a very caring missionary from Adelaide, Australia patrolled every night to be sure that all was well in the dormitories. He would frequently come down to the study hall and tell me to go to bed and get some sleep. He knew that I was determined to do well in my exams and thought I was overly industrious but he did not realize that I was suffering from serious insomnia.

Just before my board examinations were due to begin I could not sleep at all. The tension of the examinations exacerbated the situation. One night when Brother Whiting was doing his rounds, I confessed my situation to him. He realized then that I was suffering from sleep deprivation and immediately spoke to the school nurse who gave me some bitter potion to drink at bed-time. That gave me at least 3-4 hours sleep but then I would be wide awake. It was almost two weeks before the exams and I still couldn't sleep well. Brother Whiting became very concerned that I was worried that I might not perform very well in the examinations.
My first exam was physics, which I answered well (scored 91 %). At around 10 pm Brother Whiting came to my bed and gave me a neck and back massage. I'll never forget that moment

and after that I slept right through till the morning. From then on, before every examination, he would do the same for 5 to 10 minutes. It broke the cycle and gave me a vocation for life. After the examination I went to Calcutta to spend some time with my Mother. Nearly every night she would give me a massage on the neck and head. I was able to sleep normally again. Nowadays I work hard during the day with no time for reading or writing so I read and write books and articles at night. I have got into the habit of sleeping for only 4-5 hours. Often after a long flight, I ask one of my therapists in the clinic to give me a neck massage, which helps me with the jet lag.

Over the years I have developed a system of treatment for my patients which has proved immensely successful. For more than 20 years I have been taking groups of patients to the Himalayas in India for therapy. The effect of altitude, massage, yoga, and walking and diet has a tremendous impact on healing.

We usually stay in Taragarh Palace Hotel in the Kangra Valley in India. About 10 years ago, the Prince of Kashmir, who owned the Palace, was rebuilding a house within the compound that had remained unused for 60 years. Everyone had kept away as there were many stories about it being 'haunted'. I wanted to see the new house. The Prince's estate manager offered to take me there. From the first floor terrace one could get a panoramic view of the high mountains. I walked briskly to the terrace, as I was anxious to see the view. As I did so my forehead hit the beam of the door and I stumbled and fell to the floor. I saw stars, felt very dizzy, rather sick and when I tried to focus, my vision was blurred. I lay on the floor for a few minutes and then, aware of his concern, forced myself to get up slowly. I assured him that I was alright but the dizziness continued and I had to lean against the wall. I was very perplexed. How could I hit that beam? It was a normal door, the beam was above my head, so what happened? I lay in bed for the rest of that day and slept deeply until I was woken up for dinner, where the others in the group were very concerned about my injury. I had some neck pain and soreness in the forehead so I asked one of my therapists to massage my neck and put a hot salt poultice on it, after which, I slept very deeply. Next morning I woke up feeling better. There was no dizziness but a mild headache remained. Feeling somewhat weak I went downstairs for breakfast and later took a walk with the group. The dizziness gradually disappeared. The flight back home to London was comfortable but I had an unusual fatigue and the jet lag was worse that time. Then I begun to heard a continuous ringing in my right ear which was tinnitus, another symptom of the Neck Connection. I immediately began to treat my neck myself. The tinnitus went after a few days of treatment.

We never know when we will turn a corner and an event will take place that will affect our lives. Such an event happened to me one day on one of the walks on my Himalayas trips. As we took one path we were surprised to see it led to a collection of caves and beautiful waterfalls. We walked through to get to the complex. In the background behind us we could see the mighty snow-capped Himalayas and members of our party stopped frequently to take photos of the green fields with the mountains in the background. It was one of the most spectacular, interesting and impressive walks I had ever been on. We were fascinated to discover that in one of the caves there lived a Holy man. He was in his eighties, wore simple clothes and had very long hair (about 1.5 metres). Here in the cave Baba Sant Ram meditated and lived his life. He had left the British army when he was 20 years old and had moved into the complex of interconnected caves. It was here that for thousands of years other Holy or Spiritual men had lived. The paintings on the wall were evidence of past habitation. The Baba or sage was highly gifted and gave discourse on life, religion and spirituality. My visiting guests were amazed and enraptured. He asked one guest to press his left index finger with her hands then closed his eyes and told her quite accurately about her past, her circumstances and incidents that only she knew. The visitors were stunned by the visit and it was to become a regular part of my trips with patients to the Himalayas.

My Indian treks became an important part of my healing services so I decided to make a documentary film. I travelled around India interviewing various masters accompanied by a cameraman called Kedar. I interviewed the 90 year old world famous yoga master Iyengar and the 95 year old head of the Ramakrishna Mission in Belur on the bank of the Hooghly River in Calcutta. I met so many exceptional men connected with health and spirituality. During our travels we went to the Kangra valley in the Himalavas intent on filming Baba Sant Ram. We arrived at the Palace in the evening and I asked to be taken to the caves to meet the Holy Man. I had felt deeply compelled to go and visit Baba. It was a huge shock therefore when he told me that the Baba had died that very morning.

The next morning, I went to the caves to pay my last respects. Waiting there was his eldest son, Hari Singh. Who told me that his father had a premonition that I would be coming but that he would be too late. He had told his son about the bamboo bridge that I had helped to build so that the villagers were able to cross the river, especially when the water level was high. That day, on that spot, I decided to open a charity clinic for the poor people in the area. I made the announcement to the family and to hundreds of villagers that had gathered for a prayer meeting for the Baba. We walked to the waterfall, a truly peaceful place which is my paradise. As I walked down I fell sliding down the rocks. Was it an accident or a test of my intention?

A few days later, when my group arrived we went to the caves for picnic. My son Azeem was with me and as I walked from the waterfall towards the huge boulders, where everyone was having lunch, something strange happened. I fell on my back into the pool that was full of rocks. I distinctly remember hitting a rock submerged in the pool and instantaneously jerking my head forward in a reflex. That saved my head from hitting the rock. Everybody rushed towards me to pull me out of the pool. What a lucky thing that was!

What saved me was that jerking reflex that pulled my head up. Sylvester Stallone once told me that when you are knocked down in boxing match and you land on your back the most dangerous injury is sustained by the neck. Before the back of your head hits the floor it swings forward in a reflex, injuring neck muscles. It is worse than whiplash which is a horizontal movement. The neck muscles pull your heavy head up against the force of gravity.

I was shocked and had a sinking feeling and I lay on a boulder. Everybody who was there including Azeem, was shocked too. We all thought of the worst scenarios of a spinal injury. Was this a message, a test or a warning about something? Certainly the inhabitants of that unique and isolated area had no medical support. That evening I had a rare headache and felt very tired. I slept on a very thin pillow and fortunately my therapists knew what to do to the neck to prevent complications.

A month later, I was going to a friend's house for dinner and had a perfect example of the old saying 'more haste, less speed'. I was already running late because of the heavy traffic but my car needed filling so I stopped at a petrol station on the way. I filled the tank and hurried towards the kiosk to pay and as I did so, I rushed into a full-length glass door. I hit my nose badly, it bled profusely and I was shocked and dizzy. The assistant at the till was very concerned and hurried over with some tissues. After I paid the bill I went back and sat in my car for several minutes with my door open – I was dazed and my neck hurt. I pulled myself together and drove slowly to my friend's home and there I put some ice cubes on the nose to stop the bleeding.

The truth is, apart from hurrying because I was late, my mind was elsewhere. My thoughts were far away in India. I was thinking about the caves and the Baba and my proposed clinic. That very morning I had passed the last barrier. I had committed myself to opening a clinic there and the agreement to buy the plot near the caves was signed.

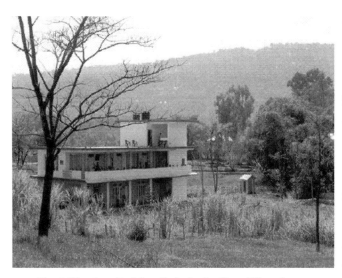

Dr Ali's charitable clinic in Indian Himalayas

My life would never be quite the same again. It had been a very special day that ended in a big neck injury. Since that day much of my heart is there underneath the magnificent Himalayas in my clinic close to the caves which has grown from nothing to a busy clinic that brings relief to the thousands of people who cannot afford good medical treatment. Everything is provided free of cost for the people of the valley.

After these three injures in a row, I became more aware of the consequences and the health risks through injuries to the neck. I began to have treatment for the neck from time to time. I now understand that I too have a neck issue and I am convinced that if I didn't take care of it I would be in trouble. I do get tinnitus when I am tired, suffer from short-term memory loss when I work non-stop for a few weeks in a row and have had blurred vision on occasion.

As a tall man I have hit my head on car doors, headboards of beds, low ceilings etc and fortunately know what to do.

I have used the neck treatment to help myself, my family and thousands of patients. The results have been amazing. My sons Shahzad and Azeem know that whenever they got a cold or cough I used the neck massage to fix their weakened immune system. I used sinus oil, vitamins and minerals and gave them breathing exercises. It always worked for them.

Recently, Shahzad went to Peru and up to Machu Pichchu and Lake Titicaca at 4000 metres with some friends. I told him to use the neck massage technique. He had always suffered from altitude sickness above 2000 metres in the Himalayas. This time, thanks to the massage treatment, he had no problem at all. His friends also didn't have any symptoms of altitude sickness, even though they were prone to it in the past.

I spend a great deal of time travelling these days. Every week I fly from my Clinic in London to Florence to treat patients in the Castel Monastero Spa, Tuscany in Italy and Forte Village, Sardinia in Italy. I also had a typical whiplash injury when I stopped at the traffic lights on Park Lane in London and a large white van hit me from the back at full force. I was jerked forward and injured my neck. It gave me a lot of pain, palpitations, fatigue and anxiety. All these affect my neck during my frequent flights. I have experienced the Ali Syndrome myself but my regular neck treatment and exercises keep everything under control. I am rarely ill with colds & flu so the immune system is strong and I have good energy.

My personal experiences of neck problems have gone a long way to convince me that my discovery, hypothesis and treatment are successful and unique. I have come to understand the matter thoroughly and can now openly discuss it with confidence and conviction.

## Conclusion

I cannot make my point about the importance of the neck more strongly than by telling you a story that touched me most deeply. It happened to one of my old school pupils. Dasgupta did very well and was promoted to a high post in the Calcutta Port Trust in India. He lived with his wife and son in a beautiful apartment and life was perfect. One day his son, while washing his face in the basin, raised his head and hit the tap. He immediately collapsed and lay unconscious on the floor. Later, his mother rushed him to the hospital but he was dead on arrival. The tap had hit the back of the child's head, jolted the tender neck and the vertebral arteries probably got compressed. The acute decrease in blood flow switched off the vital centers in the brain stem that control breathing and heart beat.

Dasgupta sold his flat and went to live with his wife in a remote village near Darjeeling in the Eastern Himalayas. He gave up his prosperous life and now dedicates his life to teaching underprivileged tribal children. I felt compelled to write this book and that story completes the circle. I started by reminding my readers that a sharp blow to the neck can be fatal and now I end with an example of that truth.

# Epilogue

It is fair to say I have discovered the role of the vertebral arteries in the neck, in health and disease. An Italian surgeon, managed to cure several cases of Multiple Sclerosis by operating on the veins of the neck. There has been a lot of press about this, following which some MS patients held pickets in Canada, outside the offices of Medical Authorities there, demanding that more research should be done to make such treatments are available there. A professor in Leeds University in the UK carried out some trials and proved that neck massages helped to lower High Blood Pressure. His explanation was that some "trigger points" in the neck had this amazing effect. I know why these results are puzzling scientists. There is a talk in Italy about carrying out Research on the neck arteries to see what else they can cure. I am glad that they are seriously looking for some clue.

I have an edge over all these scientists because not only do I know what happens when there is lack of blood flow to the brain but also know how to treat in treatment of numerous diseases with my technique. I started over 22 years ago and have tremendous experience.

Currently, I am the Head of The Clinical Spa called Castel Monastero and MITA Resort Srl, Italy near Siena in Tuscany, Italy. It is a 1100 year old Monastery converted into a beautiful 75 rooms hotel with my Clinical Spa where I run my unique Health Programmes. People come with a variety of health problems but the treatments are almost identical. They follow my diet, have my neck massage, and Marma massage (using points in the body), do yoga, drink my teas and walk or exercise and only sometimes specific remedies and supplements are used. People get cured of fatigue, headaches, backaches, digestive problems, allergies, stress, weight gain, etc and they feel and look good. It is worth bearing in mind that any massage, for example, rubbing cold hands, increases blood flow above normal, hence improvement in brain function by massaging the neck is to be expected.

I know very well that I have written a controversial book and do expect a lot of challenges to my hypothesis for which I am mentally ready. I would like to see research being carried out in future to prove that reduced blood flow to the brain can cause a variety of symptoms. PET scan is carried out by injecting radio active glucose into the blood. This injected glucose is carried by blood to various parts of the brain so its low density in an area means poor blood flow. In Chronic Fatigue Syndrome, PET scan showed general reduction of blood flow to the brain. Thus we do not have the technology to prove that minute reduction of blood flow in smaller blood vessels of the brain can cause symptoms of illness. Moreover, the tests have to be carried out when the actual symptoms are felt or recorded. If a person is dizzy, then one should record the changes in blood flow in the cerebellum as it happens and after the treatment. Headache would be a good symptom to study as it stays for a while but if blood circulation is restored (measurable) those symptoms would disappear.

I faced the humiliation of being called a masseur for extensively using my hands to treat. Often medical insurance companies refused to accept me as a provider or specialist of Complimentary Medicine and yet I have saved them hundreds of thousands of pounds every year in expensive medical treatment. Now I face the prospect of being challenged by these companies due to increase in claims by patients. I had to tell my story for the sake of millions who are suffering due to accidents, traumas, excessive computer use, stress, birth injuries etc.

# Acknowledgements

This book would not have been possible without the trust of thousands of patients who were treated by me over the years. I thank them all. I thank Ruggero Magnoni, Danish Siddiqui, The Pier2Pier team for all their help.

I want to thank Ken Bridgewater and Azeem Ali for editing this book.

I am deeply grateful to His Majesty Sultan Qaboos bin Said Al Said of The Sultanate of Oman and HRH The Prince of Wales for their constant support over the years in my work.

# Dr. Ali's Health Products

### Dr. Ali's Detox Tea

This is a blend of traditionally used herbs that helps to control excess stomach acid, suppress fungal and yeast overgrowth and restore functions of the liver. It is also used in Dr. Ali's Detox Programme and Weight Loss plan.

### Dr. Ali's Himalayan Tea

It is a blend of White tea, holy Basil, Wild mint, and Rhodedendron flowers collected at over 8000 feet by local villagers. Local people use it to prevent common ailments.

### Dr. Ali's Joint and Bone Support

A blend of vitamins, minerals and supplements, that is useful for joint and bone care.

### Dr. Ali's Women's Support

Natural supplements useful in maintaining women's general well-being

### Dr. Ali's Immune Support

A blend of vitamins, minerals and supplements useful for maintaining the balance of the Immune System.

### Dr. Ali's Energy Support

A blend of vitamins, minerals and supplements useful in boosting Energy.

### Dr. Ali's Sinus Oil

A blend of natural oils, used traditionally, to keep the nasal tract and sinuses clear.

### Dr. Ali's Joint Oil

A blend of natural oils used traditionally to help inflammation of joints and muscles.

## Dr. Ali's Back Massage Oil

A blend of natural oils used traditionally to help in soothing backache, muscle ache and tendonitis.

## Dr. Ali's Lifestyle Massage Oil

A blend of natural oils used traditionally for regular massage to relax the body and the mind.

## Dr. Ali's Junior Massage Oil

A blend of natural oils used traditionally for regular massage of babies and children.

## Dr. Ali's Elixir Vita

A blend of natural tinctures, blended with fruit juices and used as a tonic to boost energy. (Contains alcohol,)

## Dr. Ali's Elixir Nutrigest

A tonic to aid digestion made from blended natural tinctures and fruit juices. (Contains alcohol.)

## Dr. Ali's Elixir Tranquil

A blend of natural tinctures and floral extracts, used traditionally to relax the mind and body and aid sound sleep. (Contains alcohol.)

# Dr. Ali's Other Books

### *The Integrated Health Bible*

It is a book that introduces Dr. Ali's philosophy and methods of treatment.
The punch line is that the body can heel itself provided the sight conditions are set up for it to do so. It has a M.O.T. (My Own Testing) which helps you to assess your current state of health. It also has explanations for different types of diagnosis he uses (Tongue, Iridology, Pulse, Earology, Nails). The second part deals with his treatment plan for common ailments. It was on the Best Seller list in the UK.

### *Dr. Ali's Ultimate Back Book*

Dr. Ali is an expert in backache treatment. He emphasizes the sale of muscles in maintaining posture. Bad posture, traumas, repetitive strain, nutrition, insomnia, stress, auto immune disease, etc. are the main causes of backache. He discusses various types of backache and explains how they are treated, based on over 5000 cases of backache that he has seen. There are self-help methods of treatment explained very simply in the book. It sold over 35,000 in UK.

### *Dr. Ali's Nutrition Bible*

Nutrition is not about vitamins and supplements. The book goes straight into traditional knowledge. It teaches you how to select, cook and eat food. It talks about fasting therapy and its benefit. Then Dr. Ali describes the menu for different types of ailments from common cold to irritable Bowel Syndrome. UK's popular talk show "Richard and Judy" praised it live on TV.

### *Dr. Ali's Therapeutic Yoga*

This book was jointly written with a colleague at the time. Dr. Ali explained what Therapeutic

Yoga is and how it helps to cure various ailments. The yoga postures are easy to follow.

## *Dr. Ali's Weight Loss Plan*

In this book Dr. Ali explains that these are five types of weight gain. They are hormonal, dietary, psychological, genetic/familial and drug-induced. Of the causes differs, the treatment too must vary. Dr. Ali explains how each of these types can be treated.

## *Dr. Ali's Women's Health Bible*

Dr. Ali wrote a column in the *YOU* magazine of *The Mail* on Sunday in the UK. It had 3 million readers and it was the most popular health column. Its women readers asked questions and every week Dr. Ali answered them.

Dr. Ali wrote this book to answer all question on Women's Health and wellbeing. It talks about weight gain, hormonal changes, Pregnancy, Childcare, Sexual Health, Beauty, Ageing and Common diseases that women predominantly suffer from. It is another Best Seller written by Dr. Ali. It has been translated into Chinese and Italian. A great book for women.

# # #